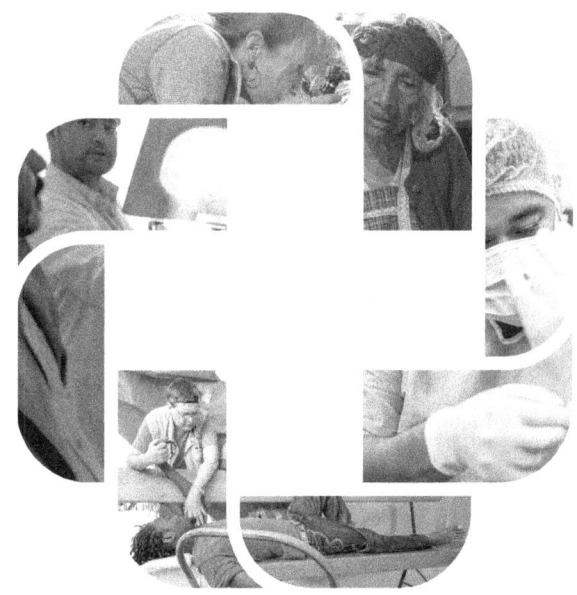

CHRISTIAN GLOBAL HEALTH IN PERSPECTIVE

A Guide to Healing and Wholeness in Missions

Rebecca Meyer, editor

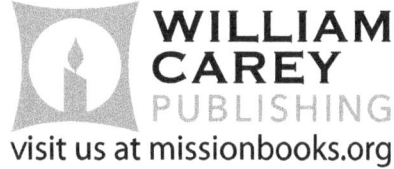

visit us at missionbooks.org

Christian Global Health in Perspective: A Guide to Healing and Wholeness in Missions
© 2024 by Frontier Mission Fellowship. All Rights Reserved.

No part of this book may be reproduced, stored in a retrieval system, or transmitted in any form or by any means—electronic, mechanical, photocopy, recording, or otherwise—without prior written permission from the publisher, except brief quotations used in connection with reviews. This manuscript may not be entered into AI, even for AI training.
For permission, email permissions@wclbooks.com. For corrections, email editor@wclbooks.com.

William Carey Publishing (WCP) publishes resources to shape and advance the missiological conversation in the world. We publish a broad range of thought-provoking books and do not necessarily endorse all opinions set forth here or in works referenced within this book.

The URLs included in this workbook are provided for personal use only and were current as of the date of publication, but the publisher disclaims any obligation to update them after publication.

Scriptures are taken from the Holy Bible, New International Version®, NIV®. Copyright © 1973, 1978, 1984, 2011 by Biblica, Inc.™ Used by permission of Zondervan. All rights reserved worldwide. www.zondervan.com. The "NIV" and "New International Version" are trademarks registered in the United States Patent and Trademark Office by Biblica, Inc.™

Published by William Carey Publishing
10 W. Dry Creek Cir
Littleton, CO 80120 | www.missionbooks.org

William Carey Publishing is a ministry of Frontier Ventures
Pasadena, CA | www.frontierventures.org

Cover and Interior Designer: Mike Riester

ISBNs: 978-1-64508-564-5 (paperback)
       978-1-64508-566-9 (epub)

Printed Worldwide

28 27 26 25 24   1 2 3 4 5   IN

Library of Congress Control Number: 2024933538

Contents

Preface v

Section 1—Biblical Foundations for Missions | Daniel O'Neill and Paul Hudson

Lesson 1—Creation, Health, and Wholeness 3

Lesson 2—The Fall, Disease, Suffering, and Death 9

Lesson 3—Salvation, Healing, and Mission 17

Section 2—Historical Foundations | Christoffer Grundmann and Paul Hudson

Lesson 4—From Jesus's Healing Ministry to the 19th Century 27

Lesson 5—Christian Medical Missions during the 19th and 20th Centuries 35

Lesson 6—Christian Global Healthcare from the 20th to 21st Century 43

Section 3—Cultural Perspectives | Rebecca Meyer and Grace Tazelaar

Lesson 7—Worldview, Culture, and Health 57

Lesson 8—Cultural Factors Impacting Health 73

Lesson 9—Culture and the Unseen World 87

Section 4—Strategic Innovation | Arnold Gorske, Rebecca Meyer, Perry Jansen, and Mike Soderling

Lesson 10—Health Promotion and Disease Prevention 101

Lesson 11—Churches, Hospitals, and Health Systems 111

Lesson 12—Leadership, Innovation, and Emerging Practices 125

Contributors 139

Preface

Welcome to the Christian Global Health in Perspective course where participants will examine health from a biblical perspective, the history of missions, cultural perspectives, and the role of the church in healthcare missions. According to Dan Fountain, "our concept of health is too short; our biomedical model of medicine is too narrow … we offer sickness care rather than health care" (1989, 1).

God's desire for health and flourishing is different than the medical model. Health from a biblical perspective relates to wholeness in body, mind, and spirit—*shalom*. To be able to help and serve people wholistically, believers need to understand God's desire for people to know him, how sin and suffering affect the world, and how the work and ministry of Jesus through his people is to be understood in this context.

The course is set up with short readings, videos, reflection questions, lectures, and online discussion sessions so that learners can walk away with tangible ways to apply the knowledge to their practice. Trained facilitators will guide the process.

Purpose of the Course

The purpose of the course is to prepare those trained in the health professions, church leaders, development workers, and other believers about the importance of God's plan for health and healing for all peoples—all *ethne*. All believers can be fully engaged in caring and showing the love of Jesus to the vulnerable because health concerns everyone.

Course Description

Participants will review the biblical basis for health in mission, the history of medical/healthcare mission, culture and worldview, and current and future global health strategies. This may result in a paradigm shift for some who view remission of disease as the sole focus for healing, when from a biblical perspective, wholeness, and the concept of *shalom* form the basis for promoting health in all its fullness. Other concepts to be explored include God's kingdom, the gospel, redemption, salvation, suffering, compassion, worldview, cultural humility, powers and principalities, health promotion, Christ-like leadership (servant leadership), and adaptive leadership.

Course Objectives

By the end of the course, participants will be able to do the following:

- Articulate important principles of biblical faith and their implications for Christian ministries of wholistic health and healing.
- Examine the ways God's people have engaged in wholistic healthcare practices throughout history to the present day.
- Compare various worldviews with a biblical worldview and how culture affects current practices of health and healing around the world.
- Plan innovative strategies for the church to promote wholistic health, healing, and restoration of *shalom* locally, nationally, and globally.

Project Contributors

There has been an excellent team of professionals who spent countless hours talking together, researching, reading manuscripts, writing content, and revising this curriculum. May it glorify the Lord to the ends of the earth. We would like to thank these consultants and advisors: Neil Thompson, E. Anthony Allen, Jacob Blair, Bruce Dahlman, Ron Halbrooks, Steve Hardy, Laura Smelter, and Willard Swartley.

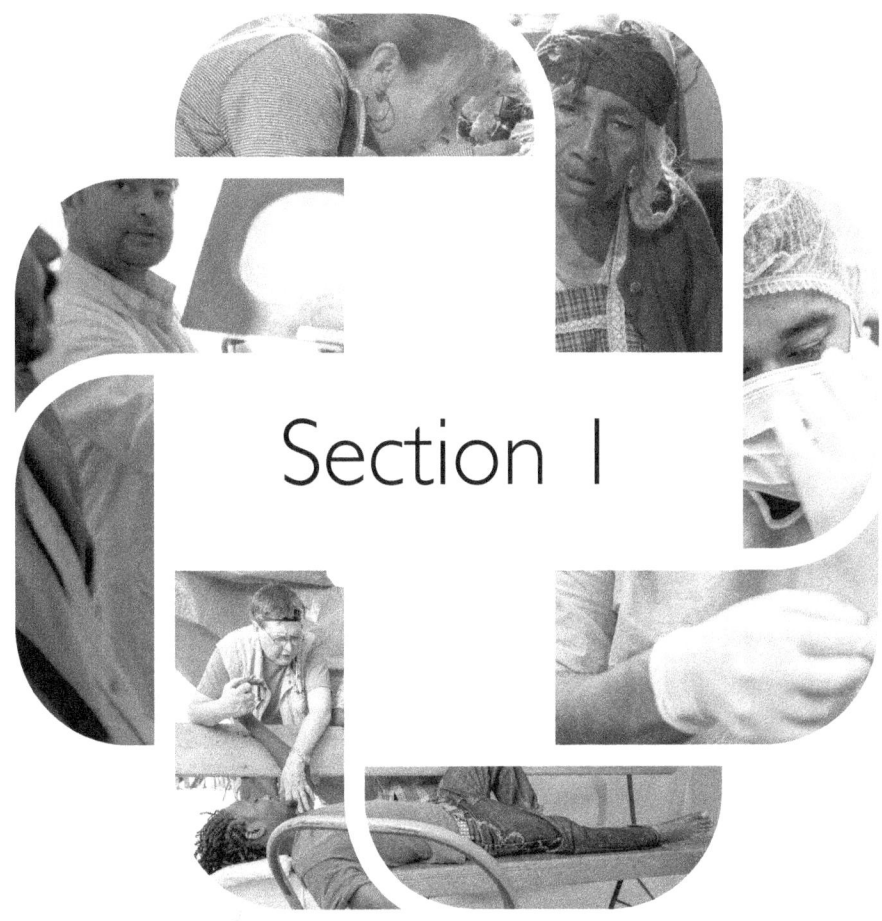

Section 1

Biblical Foundations for Missions

Daniel O'Neill and Paul Hudson

Lesson 1
Creation, Health, and Wholeness

Summary	Knowledge Objectives
God created life and desired that all people should enjoy well-being and genuine peace (*shalom*), creating order out of disorder. Jesus came that all people may have life and have it abundantly (John 10:10). In light of Jesus's mission, we as his followers can glorify God by understanding his global plan for health and well-being.	1. Identify biblical narratives for healing/mending and *shalom* and relate these to the contemporary concepts of "health" and "healing." 2. Describe health as wholeness in terms of physical well-being, one's right relationship to self, others (including enemies), God, and the environment using a biblical perspective.
Thematic Content	**Attitude Objectives**
• The creation accounts declare humans to be made "in the image of God" (Gen 1:27) and called to be productive stewards of the earth. • God declared all creation as "good," even as "very good" (Gen 1:31). • God is the ultimate healer. Health is experienced in relation to him. • Scripture gives some directions about how to live a healthy life in community.	1. Relate being made in God's image to your own personal calling and to the sacredness of human life. 2. Describe how Christians anticipate and practically realize in their own lives the hope for what ultimately will come in the end, and the hope that engenders.
Conceptual Thread—*Shalom*	**Practice (Skills) Objectives**
"*Shalom* means just relationships (living justly and experiencing justice), harmonious relationships and enjoyable relationships. *Shalom* means belonging to an authentic and nurturing community in which one can be one's true self and give oneself away without becoming poor. Justice, harmony, and enjoyment of God, self, others, and nature; this is the *shalom* that Jesus brings, the peace that passes all understanding." (Wolterstorff 1983, 69–72)	1. Identify biblical directives that promote good health and well-being, and list how these might apply to your context. 2. Create biblically informed strategies that promote comprehensive well-being in communities, and how to attribute these to God.

Part 1—*Shalom* and Relationships from Creation into Eternity

God created the universe, and there is a goodness, beauty, complexity, and healing evident in the created order. Humans are living beings made in God's image and likeness (Gen 1:27) as stewards of creation. This was retained after the fall (Gen 3:1–24) and even after the flood (Gen 9:1, 6). God declared all creation as good, and even very good (Gen 1:31) and showed the value of gender distinction, marriage, procreation, and labor. Human beings, the crowning glory of the creation, were originally given dominion over creation and access to the Tree of Life and other natural resources for health.

Adam and Eve experienced wellness, integrity, intimacy with God, wholeness, and human flourishing (*shalom*). People were made to be healthy, flourish in the beauty and complexity of the created order, work the land, and serve others while glorifying the Lord. The reason believers try to find ways to heal others, build relationships, and care for people who are not flourishing can be found in the creation narrative (Myers 2015).

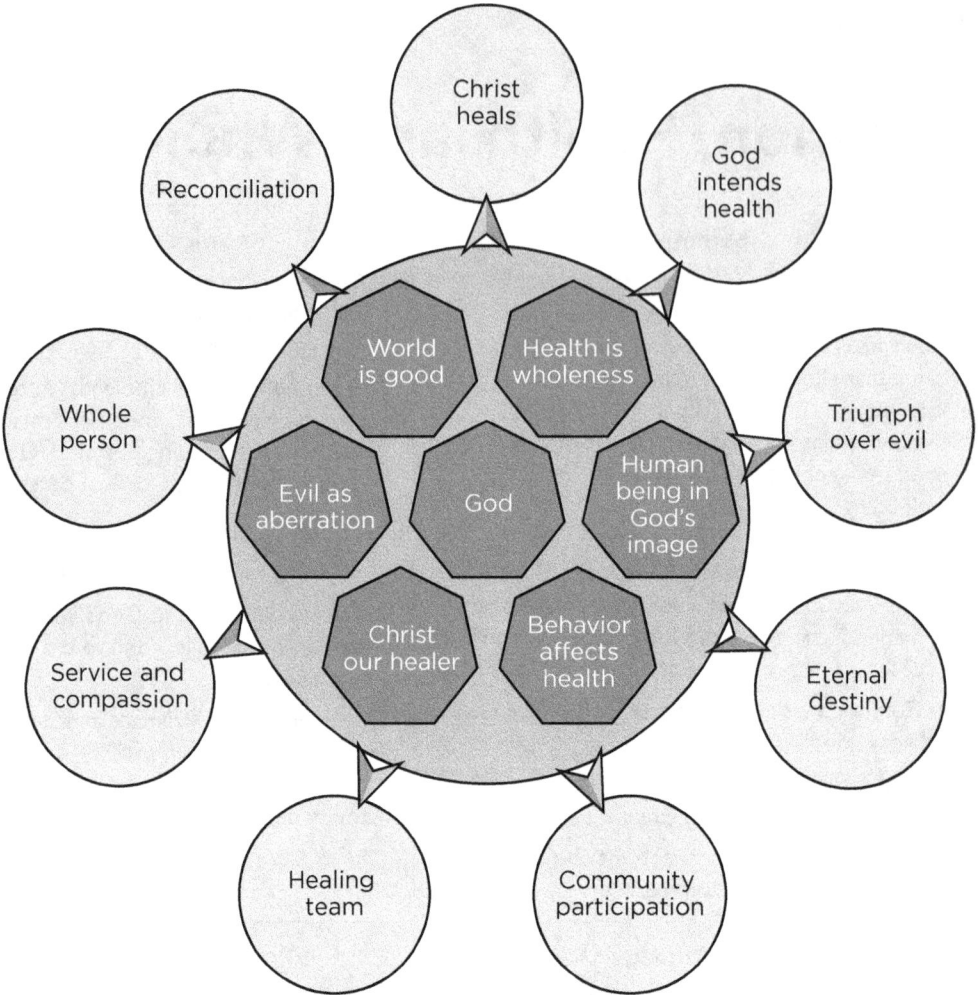

Figure 1: Thinking Biblically about Health (adapted from Fountain 1989, 51)

Adam and Eve fell into sin by rebelling against God, bringing loss of fellowship with God, disruption of *shalom*, and ultimately suffering, disease, and death (see Lesson 2). Yet even after the fall, God still plans for their redemption from sin and intends health for human beings. Christians are called to live into that eternal destiny. Health is physical well-being, but it is also related to righteousness, peace, strength, life, blessedness, holiness, and longevity. The Christian faith is a faith based on a relationship with God through Jesus Christ, and the love of Christ flows out to our relationships with people. The evil we experience is an aberration, requiring liberation, and redemption.

Broken relationships require reconciliation. A fractured self needs wholeness of body, mind, and spirit for its restoration. A disordered interaction with the natural world affects all of creation. The good news of the gospel is that God in Christ brings reconciliation with God which then brings profound healing; Jesus is the supreme healer. Hope is essential for life even in the face of certain physical death. Besides competent medical assistance, healing requires community participation and ownership. Teamwork is essential, approached with a posture of humility, service, and compassion.

Learning Activities

- **View**—Lausanne video, "Creation, Health, and Wholeness" (bit.ly/48YCBWz).
- **Read**—Genesis 1–3.
- **Review**—the graphic above "Thinking Biblically about Health."

For Those Wanting to Know More

- **Read**—Jenkins, "On Being Concerned about Medicine and Something More" (https://bit.ly/3Sif5Nr).
- **Read**—Fountain, "Thinking Biblically about Health," chapter 5 in *Health, the Bible, and the Church: Biblical Perspectives on Health and Healing*.
- **Reflect**—Fountain provides several outcomes of pursuing a biblical view of health. What other outcomes would you add? In what ways does your understanding of being healthy and being made in the image of God relate to your calling?

Part 2—Health as Restoration in Individuals and Community

As Christ-followers, one of the goals in health is bringing restoration to the whole person in community. We need science and technology as well as an understanding of the whole person in the context of their relationships. According to Dr. Daniel Fountain:

> Health cannot be defined. It is not simply an object for analysis. To render it such is to think secularly about health. Health is life, a gift we receive, an endowment we are to develop, and a journey we are to pursue. We can observe and analyze much along the way. We can manipulate and improve certain aspects of health and life. But we can never comprehend the whole…there remains a mystery. (1989, 52)

God intends humans and all creation to enjoy abundant life, of which health is a part (John 10:10). From the beginning of creation, we were designed to be in loving, just, peaceful, and enjoyable relationships. Though creation has been corrupted by the fall (Gen 3:1–20), there remains both the image of God in humans, and tremendous healing capacity in creation. Working toward health and wholeness is participating with God in his plan to restore and redeem the whole world.

God heals his people who follow his ways (Exod 15:26). The Bible gives direction about how to live a healthy life in community, though this may be only partial and temporary. Health flourishes when broken relationships to God, neighbor, self, and creation are reconciled. The "health" Christians ultimately have in mind is more than just overcoming suffering, disease, disability, and death—it is also restoring right relationships with people, planet, and God.

The Hebrew term *shalom* comes closest to representing the fullness God intends for all creation: restored wholeness, unity, justice, well-being, joy, and peace. Relationships that mirror or reflect *shalom* may also include health and fulfillment which makes the understanding of this word very relevant for this discussion. The idea of justice includes living in harmonious and enjoyable relationships. Relationships that are not just cannot be peaceful either (Myers 2009).

> *Shalom* at its highest is enjoyment in one's relationships. To dwell in *shalom* is to enjoy living before God, to enjoy living in one's physical surroundings, to enjoy living with one's fellows, to enjoy life with oneself. (Wolterstorff 1983, 70)

There are other biblical words and concepts that together give a very full meaning to health and wholeness. In addition, healing, peace, and salvation are all closely linked as God's means of restoration. Believers can align their work by cooperation with the living God. Jesus's life and work is the supreme example and means by which *shalom* and the fullness of salvation can be realized globally in individuals, communities, and nations.

Learning Activities

- **Read**—Myers, "Health, Healing, and Wholeness" (https://bit.ly/4bdoGhm).
- **Reflect**—Myers concludes that health, wholeness, and flourishing are at the center of the biblical text and is the mission of God. Why do you think this is not widely understood in churches, healthcare, or global health?

For Those Wanting to Know More

- Read the article by Christoffer Grundmann, "To Have Life and Have It Abundantly" (https://bit.ly/3IBomvU).
- Briefly summarize the biblical concepts of health presented in Grundmann's article.

Part 3—The Triune God as Ultimate Healer

All three persons of the One True God (the Trinity) are seen as healers. God's intention and actions in history are to heal a creation marred and affected by sin and Satan, the adversary. When humans fail to align with God's healing purposes, they facilitate disease and death.

There is a clear but complex relationship between faith and health. Though limited in our humanity, and mortal in our flesh, humans have been given the capacity to harness the deadly powers of nature and speak truth in order to heal. Though disease and structural evil are pervasive problems and a cause for lament, humans can experience love, healing, and peace to some degree, resulting in well-being. This was experienced in the healing Jesus brought and is represented today in the call of those sent as his ambassadors (2 Cor 5:20) and faithful witnesses.

Healing is also connected to the coming of the kingdom of God and the fall of Satan, and this ongoing work is empowered by the Holy Spirit. The church is called to be the face of healing throughout the whole world. Healing is partial now, mediated through various means, and gives opportunity to glorify God as the ultimate Healer. Striving toward healing, restoring wholeness, and fostering peace is an essential part of the mission of God. Health and healing are a foretaste of that complete health, which, finally, will be revealed to us in the consummation of the world and the renewal of all creation (Rev 21:3-4).

Seven Theses—From Scripture to Today

1. God intends *shalom* and community for humans and all creation, but sin and Satan play adversarial roles against us and God's intention for us.
2. God is God and we are weak, mortal, and frail creatures.
3. Illness puts us into a quandary before God, for it interrupts and challenges God's good world in personal experience.
4. Suffering does not mean divine absence but rather testing.
5. Jesus is Healer-Savior and leads us in faith and prayer.
6. The Spirit is Healer and is the divine pledge of complete healing.
7. The church is called to be God's face of healing in this world.

From Willard Swartley, *Seven Theses: Health, Healing, and the Church's Mission* (IVP 2012), 25-38.

Learning Activities

Read—Swartley, "Seven Theses: From Scripture to Today" (https://bit.ly/4bsyd4r).

Reflect—Develop your own list of three biblical directives that promote good health and well-being and explain how each of these might apply to your context.

For Those Wanting to Know More

Read—John Goldingay's *Theology and Healing* (https://bit.ly/3SpkbJh).

Read—Frederick Gaiser's *Healing in the Bible* (book) and reflect on these readings.

Summarize your answer to Goldingay's question: Why is a right relationship with God so important in determining well-being or health in all areas?

Reflect—Gaiser's summary includes healing as a work of God and the church as a healing community. In what ways does God act as healer through people in the world now?

References

Fountain, D. (1989). "Thinking Biblically about Health." Chapter 5 in *Health, the Bible, and the Church: Biblical Perspectives on Health and Healing*. Wheaton, IL: Billy Graham Center.

Goldingay, J. (n.d.). "Theology and Healing." https://www.gospelstudies.org.uk/biblicalstudies/pdf/churchman/092-01_023.pdf.

Grundmann, C. (2013). "To Have Life and Have It Abundantly!" *Journal of Religion and Health* 52, no. 2: 552–61.

Jenkins, D. (1981). *The Quest for Health and Wholeness*: Tubingen, German Institute for Medical Missions. https://difaem.de/fileadmin/Dokumente/Publikationen/Dokumente_AErztliche_Mission/webThe_Quest_for_Health_and_Wholeness.pdf.

Myers, B., Dufault-Hunter, E., and Voss, I. (2009). *Health, Healing, and Wholeness: Frontiers and Challenges for Christian Health Missions*. Pasadena, CA: William Carey Library.

Swartley, W. M. (2012). *Health, Healing, and the Church's Mission: Biblical Perspectives and Moral Priorities*. Downers Grove, IL: IVP Academic.

Wolterstorff, N. (1983). *Until Justice and Peace Embrace*. Grand Rapids, MI: Eerdmans.

Reflection Questions for Group Discussion

As you prepare for a time of meeting together, please prepare answers to the following questions that you can share with others:

1. How does the concept of the *Imago Dei*, the *missio Dei*, and the goodness of creation inform or affect the work that you do now?

2. What is the relationship between one's spirituality/faith and one's physical/emotional/social well-being?

3. In what ways does God act as Healer in the world?

4. What does abundant life look like in individuals? In communities? In nations?

Lesson 2
The Fall, Disease, Suffering, and Death

Summary	Knowledge Objectives
Living beings experience disease, suffering, and death which the Bible traces back to the fall. The consequence of the fall is the deprivation of the original state of wholeness and health, including fellowship with God (Gen 3). Yet, while living in a fallen world, we are sustained, often thanks to timely healing and renewal. Not every disease is healed nor is every suffering overcome and dying still must be endured. The gospel offers salvation which brings hope and meaning during the suffering we experience.	1. Describe what can be seen as consequences of the fall and how the work of Christ and his disciples leads to redemption and healing. 2. Outline different viewpoints on the problem of suffering. 3. Identify the various causes of diseases mentioned in the New Testament, including demon possession.
Thematic Content	**Attitude Objectives**
• The fall (Gen 3), separated humankind from intimacy with the living God, causing deprivations of health. • The Law (*Torah*) given to and followed by the people of God was, among other goals, meant to protect from disease and ailment (Exod 15:26). This was fulfilled in Jesus the Messiah. • Jesus Christ proclaimed the Good News of redemption from evil in word (preaching/teaching) and deed (exorcism/healing) culminating in the cross and resurrection. • Jesus Christ crucified and risen is the sole foundation for our hope for the redemption of all creation amidst injustice, disease, and suffering (1 Cor 15).	1. Locate biblical texts that describe how God reacts to the brokenness of the fallen world and reflect on what this might mean for people today. 2. Identify ways of coping that the Christian faith offers those who are suffering.
Conceptual Thread—Suffering	**Practice (Skills) Objectives**
Suffering is an experience or sensation perceived by a person as painful or harmful. It causes distress in a person's whole being, with not only physical but also spiritual, emotional, and social components. The disruption of wholesome well-being (*shalom*) at the fall led to sickness and suffering through separation from God, the Tree of Life, one another, and nature.	1. List some causes of disease and suffering in the modern world and how best to respond to them. 2. Discuss the Christian healthcare provider's role in caring for and comforting the suffering.

Part 1—The Consequences of the Fall

In the creation narratives, life-sustaining existence in the Garden of Eden was affected by the temptation of the serpent who deceived Adam and Eve by corrupting the Word of God. Thus, wholesome well-being (*shalom*) was disrupted in the fall, bringing about alienation from God, from the life-sustaining Tree of Life, from each other, and from the natural world leading to sickness, suffering, and death. The serpent and the natural environment were cursed. For humans, pain, troublesome labor (Gen 3:16–19), and disordered relationships (Gen 4:1–16) emerged, and they lost access to the Tree of

Life (Gen 3:22). This also brought about universal structural and personal evil that undermines health and well-being on a global scale up to the present day.

Disease has a multitude of causes and predisposing factors. Many of the Hebrew people of the Old Testament believed that diseases came because of sin and were a punishment from God for sin (Fountain 1989). Tracing out the etiologies can be a complex endeavor, and no one set of causes can explain all the diseases that affect people. Natural causes such as infectious agents, nutritional deficiencies or excesses, toxic chemicals, ionizing radiation, genetic mutations, and climate change are some of these intermediary causes. Unhealthy behaviors, disordered thinking, broken relationships, trauma, moral injury, poverty, oppression, meaninglessness, and sin all play a part.

Satan and other evil spirits (demons) can cause suffering, as well as corruption to material things and systems (the powers). However, there are also many afflictions which have no identifiable cause. Disease undermines human structure and function, shortens life, and can disrupt dignity, purpose, and relationships. More about this will be covered in future lessons.

Praying against, discerning, naming, avoiding, eliminating (casting out) diseases is to practice loving kindness toward neighbors. Suffering can be endured, and evil can be transformed into good through Christ. Responding to the suffering of others through active resistance against that which destroys abundant life, witnessing to the powers, expressing care and concern, and enduring suffering for the sake of others with hope and joy all reflect God's presence as a Christian calling.

Learning Activities

- **Read**—Fountain's "Coping with Suffering" (https://bit.ly/4b5e58g).
- **Fill-In**—Based on Fountain's diagram and narrative of "The Many Causes of Illness" (Figure 2 on next page), what would you add and why?
- **Reflect**—To what extent do you find the language of warfare an appropriate way to express how Christians should respond to illness or suffering?

The Fall, Disease, Suffering, and Death

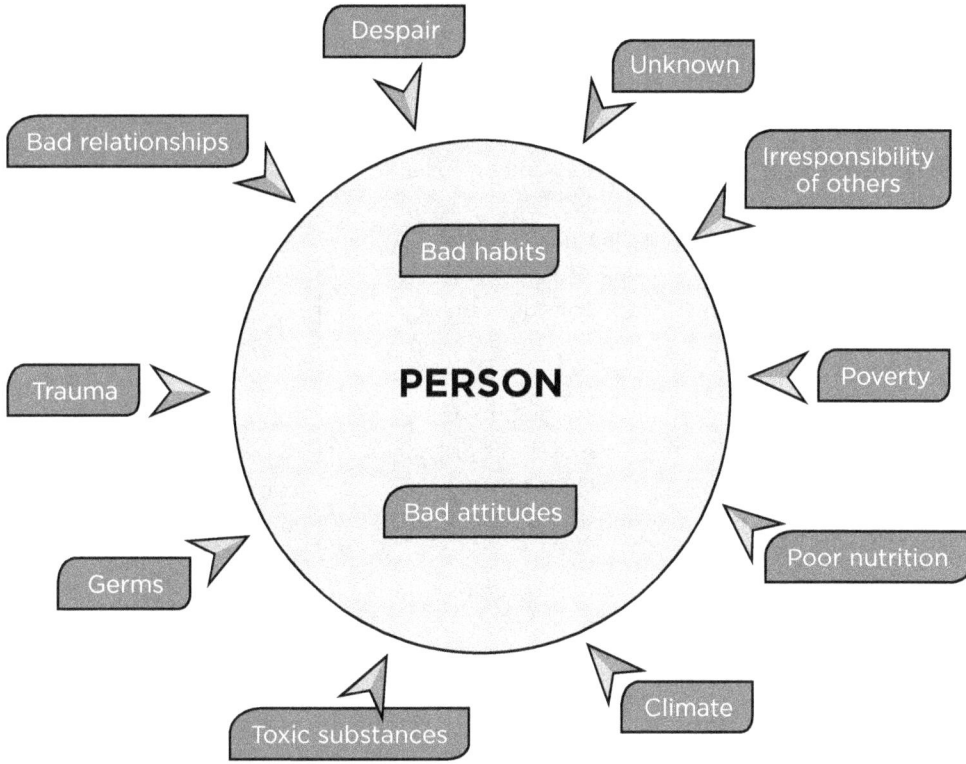

Figure 2: The Many Causes of Illness (adapted from Fountain 1989, 108)

Digging Deeper

Fountain describes how others view suffering. Fill in the blanks to complete this:

a. Dualism suggests a struggle between _____ and _____.

b. Seeing suffering as ignorance suggests that science and _____ offer the solution.

c. Fatalism suggests that suffering is just random tough _____.

d. The Bible says that although we may contribute to our own suffering, the ultimate cause of suffering is _____ , but that there is hope of strength to live by the power of _____ and hope for the future because of Jesus's _____ on the _____.

For Those Wanting to Know More

Read—T. E. Fretheim, "The Suffering of God" (https://bit.ly/3u2eKXm).

Black Death Inspires Zwingli's Plague Hymn

Ulrich Zwingli was on a mineral-springs vacation in August 1519, when the Black Death broke out in Zürich. Though weak already from exhausting work, he hurried back to his city to minister to victims. Before long he himself caught the disease and seemed likely to perish. But his work was not yet done. Zwingli recovered. His famous "plague hymn" recounts his sense of trust and then his joy at regaining health. Stanzas 1–4 were written as the disease first struck, stanzas 5–8 as his health deteriorated. Upon his recovery he finished the final four quatrains.

Stanzas 1-4	Stanzas 5-8	Stanzas 9-12
Help me, O Lord, My strength and rock; Lo, at the door I hear death's knock.	My pains increase; Haste to console; For fear and woe Seize body and soul.	My God! My Lord! Healed by the hand. Upon the earth Once more I stand.
Uplift thine arm, Once pierced for me, That conquered death. And set me free.	Death is at hand. My senses fail. My tongue is dumb; Now, Christ, prevail.	Let sin no more Rule over me; My mouth shall sing Alone to thee.
Yet, if thy voice, In life's midday. Recalls my soul, Then I obey.	Lo! Satan strains To snatch his prey; I feel his grasp; Must I give way?	Though now delayed, My hour will come. Involved, perchance. In deeper gloom.
In faith and hope Earth I resign. Secure of heaven. For I am Thine.	He harms me not, I fear no loss, For here I lie Beneath thy cross.	But, let it come; With joy I'll rise, And bear my yoke Straight to the skies.

"Black Death Inspires Zwingli's Plague Hymn." *Christian History* no. 4 (1984) (https://bit.ly/3vKgHbq).

Part 2—Finding Meaning in Illness and Suffering

Israel was given signs and the life-giving Law (*Torah*) which was intended to protect them from disease and promote societal flourishing (Exod 15:26). But this preferred state was often relinquished through disobedience. The Prophets testify to the incurable sickness brought by practicing evil ways and idolatry, and the healing that comes with repentance, faith, and obedience to the law (Jer 15:19; 17:13). Their writings express wisdom for health. "Good news and wise words are healing to the bones" (Prov 15:30; 12:18), but "cruel words are like deadly arrows" (64:3) and unconfessed sin rots the bones (Ps 32).

Sin separates and alienates people from each other, from God, and nature. Health is good, but not the ultimate good. The early church affirmed that the experience of illness awakens in the sufferer a palpable need for rescue and deliverance, but one who enjoys health and wealth can become indifferent to the need for God or indifferent toward the needs of others. Experiencing disease can be a furnace in which we are purified of our sin, weakening our disordered attachments to the empty promises of this world, and strengthening our resolve to trust God and have union with him—the ultimate Good. But suffering can also become a place of torment which de-animates, distracts, weakens, and ultimately leads to cursing God and death.

Managing disease with the former approach and rescuing from the latter response is part of a more comprehensive Christian health ministry worldwide. A Christian approach to illness always includes compassion, prayer, discernment, and truth-telling. It may also require confession and intercession, counseling, exorcism, medicine, or surgery—all for the purpose of giving glory to God and promoting health for all nations.

Learning Activities
- **Read**—Larchet's "The Spiritual Meaning of Illness" (https://bit.ly/3U8HpVk).
- **Reflect**—Larchet suggests that health can be spiritually detrimental, while illness can even constitute a blessing. How does Larchet argue this assertion?

For Those Wanting to Know More
- Read the following: John C. Thomas, *The Devil, Disease, and Deliverance* and N. G. Wright's *A Theology of the Dark Side*.
- What are the three primary causes of illness or infirmity, according to Thomas?
- List the five NT responses to illness or infirmity that Thomas suggests.
- Does any of this surprise you? If so, explain how.

Part 3—Jesus the Wounded Healer

In the Scriptures, sickness, insanity, and oppression are examples of the consequences of the fall and the effect of evil spirits. As a sign of the kingdom of God, Jesus healed those who came to him, exorcized evil spirits, and, ultimately, set people free from sin and restored them to right relationships. The crucifixion of Jesus Christ and his resurrection offers redemption for all people (and people-groups) and ultimately restoration for all of creation (Rom 8:20–22). The sacrifice on the cross leads to humanity's healing and freedom from life-destroying powers. Jesus was "pierced for our transgressions, he was crushed for our iniquities; the punishment that brought us peace (shalom) was on him, and by his wounds we are healed" (Isa 53:5 NIV) This shows the full circle of redemption of body, soul, and spirit.

Jesus as the wounded healer gives a supreme model and empowers his followers to imitate him by becoming wounded healers themselves. Christian followers are challenged to avoid the delusion of mastery of and self-sufficiency in life, and to embrace mystery and humility in the arduous task of dealing with illness. Jesus focused on individuals and crowds alike, treating each person and population as redeemable and not as a case, project, or a source of profit. He modelled composure and perseverance in the face of long days and opposition, had deep compassion, and met people where they were—addressing their felt needs. He emphasized talk and touch and taught lessons from the experience of healing. His followers become a blessing to others by imitating him, not just by engaging in health-promoting work. They expressed a sense of mercy and solidarity, with a clean heart and a spirit of reconciliation. He calls his people to live authentic lives by extending grace and being set apart for holy purposes, while at the same time acknowledging their own limitations and continual need for healing grace.

Jesus's disciples patiently bear with the sufferings of others, helping them grow, derive meaning from their illnesses, and become agents of their own healing—as co-recipients of God's grace and co-regents of God's healing work. Pastors and church leaders need not relinquish all care and concern for the body to health professionals. Health workers need not relinquish all spiritual care to pastors or chaplains given the indivisibility of the human person. The bond they create with the sufferer is fertile ground for transformation if the servants give themselves freely, listen attentively, acknowledge God's presence, and are transparent about their own humanity. In life and in death, they can be actively teaching, abiding in Christ, and sharing our Redeemer's healing love in word and deed.

> We are not the healers, we are not the reconcilers, we are not the givers of life. We are sinful, broken, vulnerable people who need as much care as anyone we care for. The mystery of ministry is that we have been chosen to make our own limited and very conditional love the gateway for the unlimited and unconditional love of God. (Nouwen 1992, 57)

Learning Activities

- **Read**—Sulmasy's "Wounded Healers" (https://bit.ly/3OksCmI).
- **Reflect**—How is it that those who are aware of their weaknesses and failures are in the best position to minister health to others as wounded healers? Why is it so important to understand the causes or meaning of one's illness?

For Those Wanting to Know More

- **Read**—Tournier's "The Mission of the Doctor" (https://bit.ly/48V9IdK).
- According to Tournier, why is it so important to understand the causes or meaning of one's illness?
- **Read**—J. Moltmann's book, *The Crucified God*, Fortress Press.
- **Reflect**—How does a theology of the cross affect your view of self-less wholistic health care?

Part 4—Offering Hope and Compassionate Care

While the redemptive work of Christ is complete through the cross and resurrection (Heb 9:12), humans live in and must endure the tension of the "already and not yet," awaiting the consummation of God's kingdom, when "God will be all in all" (1 Cor 15:28). Jesus's resurrection gives the redeemed hope for healing both now and into eternity, despite ongoing injustice, disease, disability, and suffering. The mission of Christ-followers is to bring the tangible hope of Christ's redemption and healing to the world.

The current reality of global health problems like emerging pandemics, drug resistance, ongoing extreme poverty, armed conflict, forced migration, neglected tropical diseases, increasing non-communicable diseases, gender-based violence, human trafficking, drug addiction, climate-related illness, abortion, euthanasia, and complex mental health conditions present a challenge to the church wherever it is present. These realities are also a compelling reason to send Christ-followers to demonstrate his compassion in places the church is not yet present.

One other aspect of global Christian healthcare relates to people challenged with physical, psychological, and mental impairments. More than one billion people in the world live with a disabling health condition, and most of these reside in developing countries. The biblical injunction to care for and protect the vulnerable (Isa 1:17; James 1:27), and Paul's confident trust that God's strength is made perfect in weakness (2 Cor 12:9), gives reason to see health-promoting ministries among them as intrinsic to the gospel. The disabled teach us about our common limitations, and the strength God enables. God dwells even in our brokenness and provides comfort and hope for the world. The Lausanne Covenant puts it this way:

> Although reconciliation with other people is not reconciliation with God, nor is social action evangelism, nor is political liberation salvation, nevertheless we affirm that evangelism and socio-political involvement are both part of our Christian duty. (Lausanne 2022, para 5)

Learning Activities

- **Read**—Swartley's "Disability: God's Two Hands of Love" (https://bit.ly/3vVlAhW).
- **View**—Lausanne Global Classroom, "Reconsidering Our Christian Attitude Toward Those with Disabilities" (bit.ly/3S7hxGB).
- **Reflect**—What coping mechanisms does the Christian faith offer to those who are suffering? How should the church respond to those who are suffering through marginalization, such as the blind, the lame, prisoners, the widows, orphans, and the poor?

References

Fountain, D. E. (1989). *Health, the Bible, and the Church: Biblical Perspectives on Health and Healing*. Wheaton, IL: Billy Graham Center.

Larchet, J. C. (2002). *The Theology of Illness*. Yonkers, NY: St Vladimirs Seminary Press.

Lausanne Movement. (2022). The Lausanne Covenant Statement of Faith. https://lausanne.org/content/covenant/lausanne-covenant#cov.

Nouwen, H. J. M. (1972). *The Wounded Healer*. New York: Doubleday.

Sulmasy, D. P. (1997). *Wounded Healers*. New York / Mahwah, NJ: Paulist Press.

Swartley, W. M. (2012). *Health, Healing and the Church's Mission: Biblical Perspectives and Moral Priorities*. Downers Grove, IL: IVP Academic.

Reflection Questions for Group Discussion

1. To what extent do you find the language of warfare an appropriate way to express how Christians should respond to illness or suffering?

2. Larchet suggests that health can be spiritually detrimental, while illness can even constitute a blessing. How does Larchet argue that this assertion can be true?

3. How is it that those who are aware of their weaknesses and failures are in the best position to minister health to others as wounded healers?

4. What ways of coping does the Christian faith offer to those who are suffering? How does this differ from other faiths?

5. How should the church respond to those who suffer through marginalization, such as the blind, the lame, the prisoners, the widows and orphans and the poor?

Lesson 3
Salvation, Healing, and Mission

Summary	Knowledge Objectives
The Christian mandate is to witness to God's abundant love in Jesus Christ for all people globally. Christians are invited to participate in God's healing work by proclaiming and witnessing to the Good News in both word and deed. Health workers realize this calling not just by their medical expertise but by following the Savior, who "heals the nations" (Rev 22:2) and restores *shalom*. In becoming instruments of healing, they witness to the corporeality of salvation in Christ for the whole world.	1. Identify the call of the people of God and relate that call to healthcare and health-related development. 2. Discuss Jesus's healings and how they served to proclaim the kingdom of God, citing specific Scriptures. 3. Describe what it meant for Jesus to say that the kingdom of God is near and how that relates to healing.
Thematic Content	**Attitude Objectives**
• All authentic healing is from God. • Healing is a sign of grace from God for sustaining a fallen creation. • Jesus proclaimed the kingdom of God and healed in various ways—by touch, by word, by promise, and by means. • The disciples were called and sent to do likewise (Matt 10:7–8; Mark 16:15–18; Luke 10:9) but experienced failure at times (Matt 17:19–20). • God's people are called to proclaim the good news of salvation/healing, becoming a blessing to all nations. • People of the new covenant, the church, are called to imitate Christ and to continue his ongoing ministry of healing.	1. Reflect on the various Christian viewpoints on healing, including miraculous healing and exorcism. 2. Discern how God is calling people with their specific gifts, skills, passions, and expertise to bring about healing.
Conceptual Thread—Healing	**Practice (Skills) Objectives**
Healing is experienced when broken and weak bodies are mended and regain strength. But healing is also experienced when life-giving relationships between God, neighbor, self, and creation are reconciled. However, abundant life which Christ came to bring can be realized even without full bodily recovery, even in the midst of disease and suffering. God's people are to exercise thoughtful dominion to promote health as a witness to God's healing work.	1. Discuss the church's vital role for healing in the modern world. 2. List specific ways a local church can serve the health needs of its community. 3. Describe ways to integrate medical intervention, care, and prayer.

Part 1—Creation, God's People, and Health

All healing is a work of God, and an expression of his grace. God's people are called to join in the mission of God as witnesses to God's redemptive work for the healing of all creation. The creation mandate was to steward (have dominion over and care for) the earth and oppose life-destroying powers (Gen 1:28). However, humans are made of the dust, and susceptible to frailty and subject to death (Gen 3:19; Ps 90:5–6).

There is also a clear association between human moral choices and human and planetary flourishing. Two thirds of the psalms are laments for illness, sin, calamity, or injustice, but many of these also indicate hope for healing and even overcoming death. Besides being seen as bodily afflictions, sickness is understood as a deprivation of *shalom* and right relationships.

In the Abrahamic covenant Israel was "blessed to be a blessing" to all nations/peoples, and the Messiah was to become the ultimate blessing. The covenant community of Israel emphasized health-promoting laws (Exod 19–20; Lev 11–26), and the conditional blessing of life and health through obedience to the Lord who heals (*Yhwh-rapha*, Exod 15:26). The Ten Commandments and associated Mosaic laws provide a means by which God bestows the blessing of health and healthy relationships to his people, creating preventive community structures which promote human flourishing. This was unique among the cultures of the Ancient Near East but was often hindered by human rebellion and sin.

The prophets called people to healing, and back to God's heart. Wicked ways are seen to be directly connected in a causative way to afflictions of "sword, famine and plague" in the prophets (Ezek 6:11). Prophets are held accountable for not warning people of afflictions to come (Ezek 3:18; 33:8). In contrast, blessings, peace, and renewal of the land are contingent upon righteous obedience to the law that gives life (Ezek 18:31–32). Salvation and healing are closely linked, both tied to the grace of God. A false alternative is the prosperity gospel, which makes healing a reward for believing. Old Testament scholar Christopher Wright puts it this way: "The great Christ-centered, cross-centered redemptive truths do not nullify—rather, they *complete*—all that the Old Testament revealed about God's commitment to the wholeness of human life and redeeming his whole creation, for God's own glory in Christ" (Wright 2009, para. 9).

Learning Activities

- **Read**—W. Swartley's "Healing in the Old Testament" (https://bit.ly/49eQJv9).
- **Reflect**—What elements would you add to Swartley's diagrams below: "Life devoid of Shalom" and "Life filled with *Shalom*."

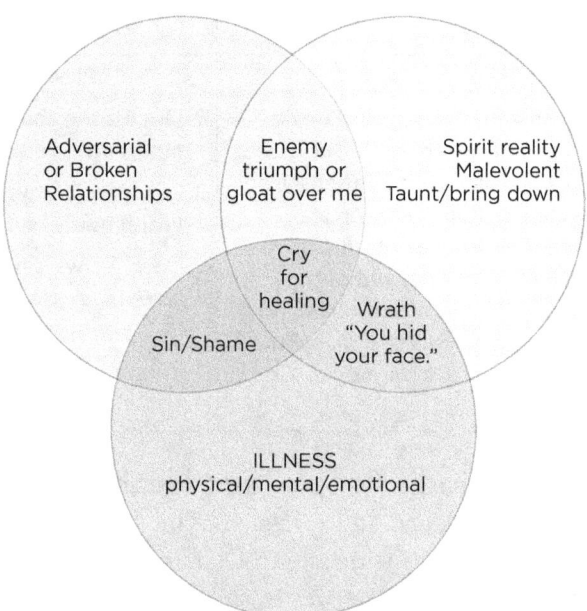

Figure 3: Life Devoid of *Shalom* (adapted from Swartley 2012, 52)

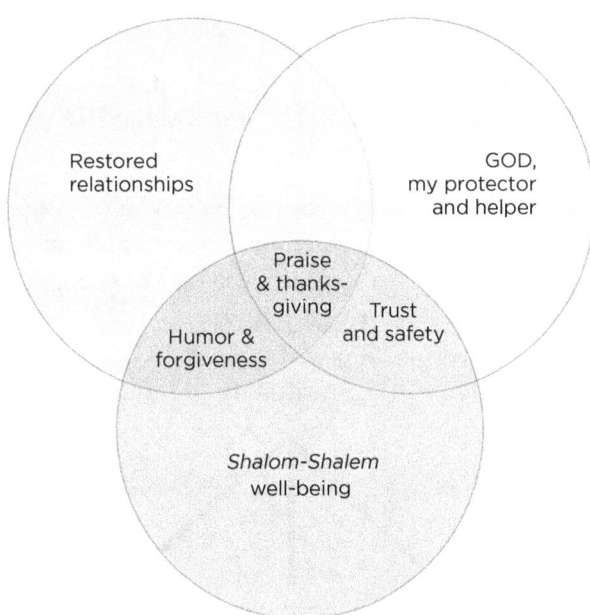

Figure 4: Life Filled with *Shalom* (adapted from Swartley 2012, 53)

Part 2—Jesus and the Ministry of Healing

Jesus fulfilled Isaiah's messianic prophecy for healing and integral mission (Luke 4:14–30). He healed and proclaimed the kingdom of God, by touch, by word, by promise and by means—leading to healing and restoration of right relationships (physical, social, spiritual, etc.). Jesus expressed compassion toward the sick, anger toward those who obstructed healing (Mark 3:5), and non-discriminating care to all those in need regardless of their social status, gender, belief, or race. He extended his healing to Romans, Samaritans and Canaanites who expressed faith, reflecting his heart for the healing of all nations (Matt 15:24–28).

Jesus went among the people, touched the unclean, and did not ignore any who did not seem to fit his agenda (Mark 5). He used healing as a lesson to teach spiritual truths to onlookers and used healing the sick as a context when he delivered his greatest sermon (Luke 6:17–22). He closely integrated healing, and proclamation of the gospel of the kingdom. He liberated others from destructive powers as signs of his divine authority and of the coming of the kingdom of God.

Jesus sent his disciples to do likewise by imitating him in compassion, service, healing, truth-telling, naming and confronting the powers, setting free, and proclaiming the Good News (Matt 10:7–8; Mark 16:15–18; Luke 10:9; John 20:21). However, the disciples did not always succeed (Matt 17:19–20). They had to learn that the power to heal was not theirs. They were sent to witness to the power of the living God in Jesus. They were later empowered by the Holy Spirit at Pentecost, and filled by the Spirit, unified in purpose, diversified in gifting, and directed to discern and confront all powers opposed to Christ.

Throughout church history, various practices of healing have persisted, witnessing to the fullness of the gospel. This includes authentic presence, proclamation, purging, and healing—life, word, sign, and deed. An effective witness often begins with loving acts which provokes questions to which the gospel is the ultimate answer. The gospel also instills the hope of healing through freedom from all powers—supernatural and natural—that destroy life. In Christ, personal integrity is restored, and *shalom* is experienced even if cure is not. Jesus as Messiah brings redemption to all creation and to all people-groups through his people.

Learning Activities

- **Read**—B. Myers' "Announcing the Whole Gospel" (https://bit.ly/47FVfBG), and Lausanne's "Whole Gospel, Whole Church, Whole World" (bit.ly/48Xhc00).

- **Reflect**—Considering Myers' graph below, "The Whole Gospel of Jesus Christ," which aspect(s) do you think need strengthening in your life and work, and what steps will you take to strengthen them?

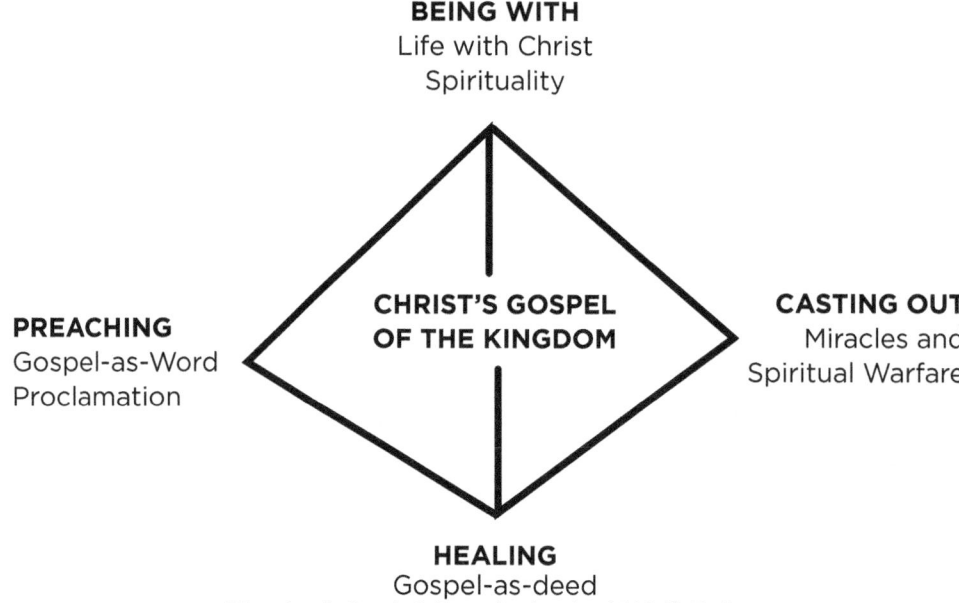

Figure 5: The Whole Gospel of Jesus Christ (adapted from Myers 2011, 101)

- **Reflect**—From your perspective, why is it that we see such a separation between those who preach and teach and those who work towards health and healing?

Part 3—The Mission of the Church

All disciples are called to have special concern for the poor, vulnerable, sick, and foreigners, and to practice justice while also witnessing to the gospel of Jesus Christ. The divine call can be expressed in four "Great C's":

- **Great Creation Mandate**—stewarding wisely the created order (Gen 1:28; 2:19).
- **Great Commandment**—loving God fully and loving neighbor fully (Matt 22:37–40; Mark 12:30–31; Luke 10:26–28).
- **Great Commission**—making disciples of all peoples, baptizing and teaching (Matt 28:18–20; Mark 16:15–16).
- **Great Convergence**—attending body, mind, soul, and spirit in both word and deed (1 Thess 5:23; Heb 4:12; 3 John 1:2).

This requires some critique of the body-mind dualism and reductionism present in Western thinking, and a return to a biblical view of the unity of the human being in the context of the community and planet to recover an effective approach to transformative healing for the church, community, and healthcare systems.

Genuine hope provides a vital perspective for all those who live in despair including those who are sick and suffering. Healthy relationships bring healing to those who are lonely or oppressed. Experiencing salvation from sin makes people whole, even if their physical vulnerabilities remain. Recognizing and opposing the spiritual powers behind some diseases and addressing corruptions in systems, praying for release from these powers, and maintaining hope for healing beyond the physiologic capacity of medicine, is moving in the power of the Holy Spirit and pursuing the hope of liberation. This requires a vision for the whole church proclaiming and demonstrating the whole gospel to the whole world—for the whole person.

By engaging the world's brokenness with demonstrations of God's loving kindness and justice, Christian global health services become instrumental in building bridges across cultures and collaborating for transformational development. As ministers of reconciliation contextualize the fullness of the gospel and interact with suffering communities, abundant life can be realized, and God can be glorified as ultimate Healer. The church, thereby, bears witness to the corporeality of salvation in Jesus Christ. Disciples recognize the temporal and only partial nature of health and healing, and the possibility of surrendering health or fortune for the sake of others and the kingdom. Yet they are emboldened by an eschatological view of the hope of complete healing for all the nations (Rev 22:2).

Learning Activities

- **Read**—E. A. Allen, "Healing the Whole Person" (https://bit.ly/3U8bJ2e), and D. O'Neill, "Theological Foundations for an Effective Christian Response" (https://bit.ly/3vLUEkI).

- **Reflect**—Allan suggests that the whole person involves not only the physical body, but a psychological, social, and spiritual dimension. From your perspective, where does most medical practice fall short in dealing with the whole person? Where does the church's spiritual ministry fall short of this whole gospel approach?

- **Reflect**—O'Neill emphasizes the biblical foundations of truth-telling, caring, peace-making, collaboration, and prioritization. List three ways in which Christians could more fully participate in reconciling all aspects of humanity among all peoples to God.

For Those Wanting to Know More

- **Read**—Joni Eareckson-Tada and Steven Estes, *When God Weeps: Why Our Sufferings Matter to the Almighty*.

References

Allen, E. A., Luscombe, K., Myers, B., and Ram, E. (1991). *Health, Healing, and Transformation; Biblical Reflections on the Church in Ministries of Healing* and *Wholeness*. Monrovia, CA: World Vision International, MARC.

Eareckson-Tada, J., and Estes, S. (1997). *When God Weeps: Why Our Sufferings Matter to the Almighty*. Grand Rapids: Zondervan. Appendix A: Scriptures on God's Hand in Our Sufferings and Appendix B: God's Purpose in Our Sufferings, 219–40.

Fountain, D. E. (1989). *Health, the Bible, and the Church: Biblical Perspectives on Health and Healing*. Wheaton, IL: Billy Graham Center.

Fretheim, T. E. (1984). *The Suffering of God: An Old Testament Perspective*. Minneapolis, MN: Fortress Press.

Larchet, J. C. (2002). *The Theology of Illness*. Yonkers, NY: St Vladimir's Seminary Press.

Myers, B., and Dufault-Hunter, E. (2015). *Health, Healing, and Shalom: Frontiers and Challenges for Christian Healthcare Missions*. Pasadena, CA: William Carey Library.

O'Neill, D. W. (2016). "Theological Foundations for an Effective Christian Response to the Global Disease Burden in Resource-Constrained Regions." *Christian Journal for Global Health* 3, no. 1: 3–10. https://doi.org/10.15566/cjgh.v3i1.112.

Sulmasy, D. P. (1997). *The Healer's Calling. A Spirituality for Physicians and Other Health Care Professionals*. New York: Paulist Press.

Swartley, W. M. (2012). *Health, Healing and the Church's Mission: Biblical Perspectives and Moral Priorities*. Downers Grove, IL: IVP Academic.

Thomas, J. C. (2011). *The Devil, Disease, and Deliverance: Origins of Illness in New Testament Thought*. Cleveland, TN: CPT Press, 296–309.

Tournier, P. (2012). Chapter 22, "The Mission of the Doctor." In *A Doctor's Casebook in Light of the Bible*. Rev ed.,178–87. Norwich, UK: Hymns Ancient Modern Ltd.

Wright, C. H. (2009). *Whole Gospel Church, Whole World*. Lausanne content library. https://lausanne.org/content/whole-gospel-whole-church-whole-world.

Wright, N. G. (2010). *A Theology of the Dark Side: Putting the Power of Evil in Its Place*. Eugene, OR: Wipf and Stock, 165–79.

Reflection Questions for Group Discussion

As you prepare for a time of meeting together, please prepare answers to the following questions that you can share with others:

1. What were some of the main biblical ideas that impacted you from this lesson? Why?

2. What did it mean when Jesus said that the kingdom of God was near? Is there a relationship between the kingdom of God and healing? If so, explain.

3. Global health ministry is central to the biblical call to participate in cooperative efforts with God to promote human flourishing. In what ways does your calling and work help people and the planet to flourish? How are you challenged to deepen that call?

4. What are the various ways the church is called to healing in the modern world? List and be prepared to discuss how a local church and faith-based organizations can follow biblical patterns to serve the health and wholeness needs of their communities.

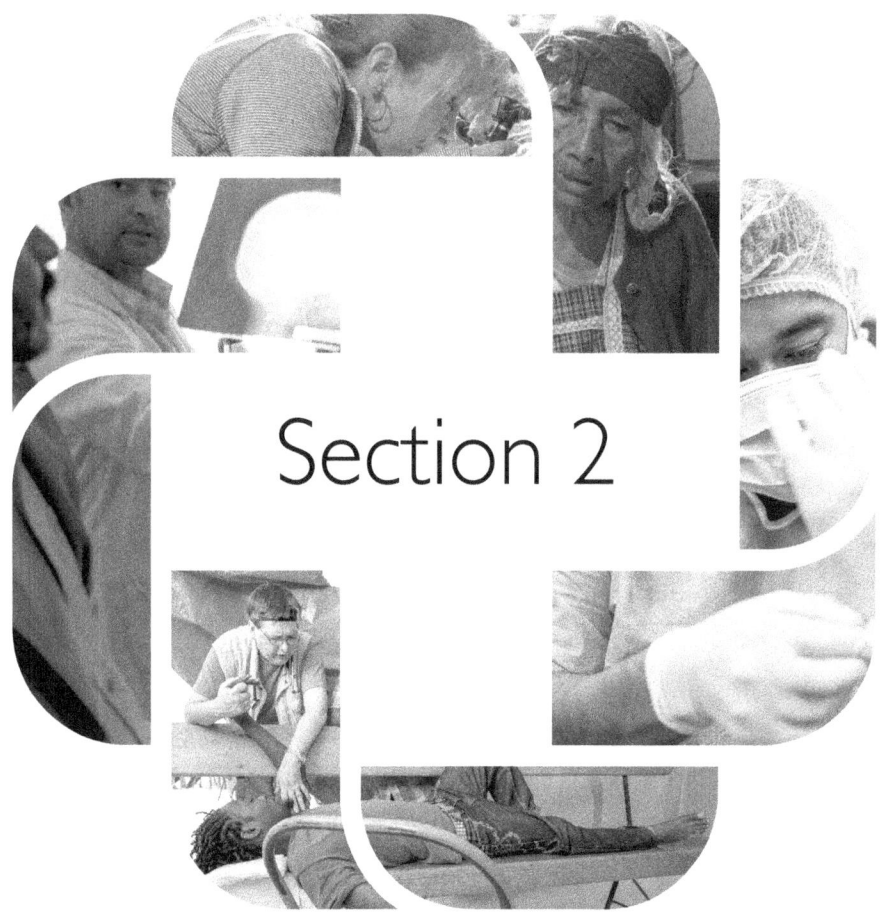

Section 2

Historical Foundations

Christoffer Grundmann and Paul Hudson

Lesson 4
From Jesus's Healing Ministry to the 19th Century

Summary	Knowledge Objectives
Jesus healed and restored people to health. He also commissioned his disciples to do likewise. The Apostles, however, had also to experience failure. Later, the church established hospitals to care for the sick and needy. Compassionate care for the diseased became thus the signature mark of the Christian healing ministry until the nineteenth century.	1. Describe the healings performed by Jesus and describe the various ways in which they were brought about. 2. List the healings done by the Apostles. 3. Name the motivation for caring for the sick in the Middle Ages.
Thematic Content	**Attitude Objectives**
• Jesus healed in various ways: by word, by touch, by means, by exorcism. • Jesus also commissioned his disciples to heal. • The Apostles healed people, but they also experienced failure. • The early church instituted the ministry of deacons and elders to visit the sick, to lay hands on them, and to pray with them. • As early as the 4th century, Christians built institutions for the care of the sick and needy (hospitals/hospices). • In the Middle Ages (8th–15th century) compassionate care for the sick by visitation at home, and in institutions (hospices/hospitals) was organized by either religious orders, civil societies, or local communities. • Male religious orders of Hospitallers charged with the care of the sick in hospitals were founded in the High Middle Ages (12th–14th century). Female orders dedicated to the same ministry followed later. • The ministry of Deaconesses was re-instituted in the church in the early nineteenth century by Theodor Fliedner at Kaiserswerth, Germany.	1. Share similarities and differences between Jesus's healing and modern medical therapy. 2. Imagine being one of the Apostles carrying out the ministry of healing in a time without modern medical means. 3. Visualize being in a hospital during the Middle Ages and how it might feel different to staying in a modern hospital today.
Conceptual Thread—Compassion	**Practice (Skills) Objectives**
Jesus Christ healed people who were sick and incapacitated in various ways. He was moved by compassion and the proclamation of the kingdom of God. His disciples are called to do likewise, even when unable to cure diseases. Christian concern for the sick and needy led to the establishment of respective institutions like hospitals and hospices. Thus, compassion in solidarity with the needy became the hallmark of Christian healthcare.	1. Articulate the difference between Jesus's healings and all other attempts at healing undertaken by Apostles, medical professionals, or spiritual healers. 2. Verbalize the early church's understanding of salvation and healing, how they overlap and where they differ. 3. Demonstrate competence in critically discerning salvation from healing.

Introduction to the History of Medical Missions

Acquaintance with the history of Christian medical missions (today known as Christian global healthcare ministries) helps to better understand the challenges these ministries face today, why they are carried out the way they are, and how they express Christian identity. History also shows how the Christian concern for global health came about, what it is rooted in, motivated by, and how its focus shifted in the course of time in response to changing circumstances.

We discern three different stages in the development of these ministries which conveniently account for the three following lessons. We describe these stages as: (1) Origins and Infancy: Jesus's healing ministry, the Apostles' charge, and compassionate care (covering the period from the time of Jesus all through the nineteenth century); (2) The time of Adolescence: Christian Medical Missions during the nineteenth and twentieth centuries; and (3) Growing into Maturity: Christian Global Healthcare in the twenty-first century.

Part 1—Healing in the Ministry of Jesus

All four gospels witness to Jesus's healing activities. While the New Testament tells of more than forty healings of individuals and groups by Jesus, the actual number was certainly higher as accounts like Matthew 9:35 suggest: "Jesus went about all the cities and villages ... curing every disease and every sickness" (see also Matt 12:15–22; 19:2; 21:14; Mark 3:10; Luke 6:18–19).

The simple fact that Jesus healed—unlike Moses or the Buddha, Confucius, Lao Tzu, or Mohamed—indicates that to Jesus, salvation unquestionably had a bodily dimension. In Jesus's ministry, healing became a legitimate corporeal aspect of salvation, though never synonymous with salvation (see Mark 2:1–12; Luke 5:17–26). In Jesus's unique ministry, physical healing often accompanied salvation. Jesus cared for people in bodily distress as an expression of his proclamation of the good news of the kingdom of God, the gospel (see also Rev 21:4; 22:2).

However, to call Jesus a "healer" or even a "faith healer," would miss the point, because in Jesus's ministry healings were just the corporeal expression of the central message that in him the "kingdom of God has come near" to mankind (see Mark 1:15; Matt 4:17). Further, Jesus did not heal by observing one established procedure. Rather, he healed in various ways: by word, by touch and being touched, by means, and by exorcism (for details see Lesson 3 of this course). Most of the people Jesus healed were in his proximity, but some he healed from a distance (see Matt 8:5–13; 15:21–28; Mark 7:24–30; Luke 7:11–10). Also, Jesus healed without a hidden agenda or desire for remuneration. And, unlike so-called "faith healers," Jesus did not always ask for faith by those seeking his help.

While there are several instances where Jesus alluded to faith (Matt 8:22; 9:27–33; Mark 5:34; Luke 7:50; John 5:1–9), there are other healings not occasioned by faith at all (Matt 8:14–15; 12:9–13) but by Jesus's compassion for the suffering instead (Matt 9:35–36). Further, many of those who Jesus healed did not become his disciples; one example of this is the healing of the ten lepers (Luke 17:11–19), a story which shows that only a fraction of those healed realize whom ultimately to thank.

Part 2—The Apostles Are Commissioned to Heal

Jesus healed by the authority of God incarnate. But he also commissioned his disciples to do likewise (Matt 10:7–8; Luke 10:9) by asking them to faithfully bear witness to God's healing power. But despite their well-intended attempts at healing, the Apostles also experienced failure (Matt 17:14–20; Mark 9:14–29; Luke 9:37–43). This experience made them realize the decisive difference between their ministry and that of their Lord and Master.

The Apostles always healed "in the name" of Jesus Christ (Mark 16:17; Acts 3:6). They came to understand that they could not avail of that name as a potent magic formula. Their power rested entirely on their own authentic believing God's promise. Thus, we see Peter and Paul bringing about healing (Acts 5:12–16; 8:6–7; 9:17; 14:8–10; 19:12; 28:8). We also learn from Paul's first letter to the Corinthians that the gift of healing was present within the early Christian community (1 Cor 12:9). We can also discern efforts at organizing a diaconal, that is, a caring ministry for needy people (Acts 6:1–6), and the visitation and anointing of the sick for healing beyond one's kin very early in the emergence of the Christian church (James 5:13–16).

Learning Activities

- **Read**—"Health and Healing in the New Testament" in: R. L. Numbers, D. W. Amundsen, eds., *Caring and Curing*, 43–60.
- **Reflect**—on the meaning of health and healing. How did Jesus heal? Whom did he heal? What was so different about the ways he healed?
- **Fill in**—the table below.

After completing the reading, describe how Jesus healed, how the Apostles obeyed the healing mandate, and how medical professionals and spiritual or traditional healers go about their work.

Jesus healed in this way	The Apostles healed in this way	Medical doctors heal in this way	Spiritual and/or traditional healers heal in this way

Answer the following questions afterward:

1. What are specific differences between the various types/methods of healing listed above?
2. What are the motivations behind Jesus's healings?
3. What are the motivations behind the Apostles' healings?
4. What are the motivations behind engaging in healing by medical professionals?
5. What are motivations behind the various healing rituals by spiritual or traditional healers?

Part 3—Compassionate Care Becomes the Signature of Christian Healthcare

While there is some evidence that Christians also cared for sick people who were not members of the church even before Christianity became a legal—and later a privileged—religion in the Roman Empire in the fourth century (313/380), it is only around that time that publicly noticeable Christian institutional care for the needy emerged. It found expression in the establishment of "hospitals" called *Xenodochia* (guesthouses) or *Nosokomeion* (refuge for the sick). These were not hospitals in the modern sense. Rather, they were decent shelters for those needing help due to lack of family or community support. We know of such institutions in Caesarea (today's Kayseri in Cappadocia, Turkey), Edessa (now Sanliurfa/Urfa, Turkey) founded in 375, Antiochia (now Antakya, Turkey; founded before 398), and Ephesus (close to today's Selçuk, Turkey) founded in 451. The most famous *Xenodochion* was the "Basilias" at Caesarea established by Bishop Basil the Great (329–79) in about 370.

Far from taking in all who needed help due to limits of space and personnel, only some of those cared for were sick. Others were orphaned or widowed, people with leprosy, or just foreigners on a pilgrimage. A contemporary of Basil who visited the Basilias, which consisted of several buildings, reported the following:

> Go forth a little from the city [that is, Caesarea/Kayseri], and behold the new city, the treasure-house of godliness ... in which disease is investigated and sympathy proved... . We have no longer to look on the fearful and pitiable sight of men like corpses before death, with greater parts of their limbs dead [from leprosy], driven from cities, from dwellings, from public places, from watercourses ... Basil it was more than anyone who persuaded those who are men not to scorn men, nor to dishonor Christ the head of all by their inhumanity towards human beings. (Gregory of Nazianzus, *Oratio* 20)

Learning Activities

- **Read**—Amundsen and Ferngren's "The Developing Church, Circa 100–400 C.E." (https://bit.ly/423fPe3).
- **Read**—Box 1, below.
- **Reflect**—on the meaning and purpose of medical care considering how Christians attended the sick and needy during the days of the early church.

> **BOX 1**
> Although their numbers and resources might be small, Christians were equipped even in the most adverse circumstances, to undertake considerable charitable activity on behalf of those who were ill. Owing to a combination of inner motivation, self-discipline, and effective leadership, the local congregation created in the first two centuries of its existence an organization, unique in the classical world, that effectively and systematically cared for the sick … The diaconal model of philanthropy was well suited to the first three centuries of Christianity, when the urban congregation was the focal point of the movement.
>
> I suggest that it was the great plague of the mid-third century [the so-called "Cyprian Plague" raging the Mediterranean countries from about 250–70] that provided the church with its greatest opportunity for the broad extension of medical charity. Its ministry to the sick had hitherto been inwardly directed, largely to its own adherents. Increasingly Christian healthcare became outwardly focused, now enlarged to include many who were victims of the plague. The administrative structure was already in place … The evidence suggests that for the first time the church conceived of its ministry to the sick as one that included both pagans and Christians without distinction. (Ferngren 2014, 114 and 121)

Part 4—Emergence of Professional Healthcare and Nursing

While healthcare and nursing in the modern technical sense were still centuries away, we can trace their beginnings back to the monastic Rule of St. Benedict (6th cent.). The Rule made care of sick brothers part of the duties of charity required of all monks.

> Care of the sick must rank above and before all else, so that they may truly be served as Christ, who said: "I was sick and you visited me" (Matt 25:36), and "What you did for one of these least brothers you did for me" (Matt 25:40)… . Sick brothers must be patiently borne with, because serving them leads to a greater reward… . Let a separate room be designated for the sick and let them be served by an attendant… . The sick may take baths whenever it is advisable … Moreover, to regain their strength, the sick who are very weak may eat meat … The abbot must take the greatest care that … those who serve the sick do not neglect them.
> (*Rule of St. Benedict* 1975, chap. 36)

Other early traces of healthcare and nursing are detectable in the founding of religious orders of Hospitallers during the tenth to fifteenth centuries. These were congregations of laymen, established by local grandees and dignitaries as meritorious works of charity in gratitude for blessings received—like a miraculous healing, for making a fortune or for safely returning from battle—and counting on eternal reward. They founded "hospitals," which on average accommodated not more than twelve individuals. These societies also secured maintenance of the place by providing nurses for the care of patients and means for its upkeep.

The first of these orders we know of are the "Hospital Brothers of St. Anthony" (Antonines) founded in France in 1095. Its members attended to sick people, particularly those afflicted with St. Anthony's fire (*ergotism*), an ailment very common among the poor in the Middle Ages. Other similar orders were affiliated with "Holy Spirit"/"Holy Ghost" hospitals built by civil authorities which flourished in many cities in medieval Europe. The most famous among those organizations is the "Order of the Holy Ghost" ("Hospitallers of the Holy Spirit") also established in France in 1161.

Mention needs to be made of several chivalric orders instituted by crusaders to attend to their comrades wounded in battle and to care for pilgrims to Jerusalem like the Knights Hospitallers (Hospitallers of St. John 1099), the Knights of the Holy Sepulcher (1099), the Order of Saint Lazarus of Jerusalem (Leper Brothers of Jerusalem/Lazarists 1119), the Knights of Saint Lazarus (1123), and the Teutonic Order (1192). The non-chivalric Brothers Hospitallers of St. John of God (Fatebenefratelli/Brothers of Mercy) devoted to the care of the sick came about much later, namely in 1572, followed by the Ministers to the Sick (Camillians/Clerics Regular) in 1582.

Female congregations dedicated to the care of the sick came into existence even later. This was due to restrictions of convent life prohibiting work outside cloistered walls. However, as early as the twelfth century lay people, female as well as male, inspired by an ideal of apostolic living in imitating Christ, devoted themselves to prayer and good works without taking vows but living celibately in voluntary poverty. The males were called "Beghards" and the females "Beguines" who far outweighed their male counterparts in number and popularity. Much of their charitable work consisted in visiting the sick in their homes and tending the needy; Elizabeth, Princess of Hungary, and Landgravine of Thuringia (1207–1231), became one of the most famous among such women. To honor her legacy the nursing order of the Hospital Sisters of St. Elizabeth was founded in 1622, while the Company of the Daughters of Charity (Daughters of Charity/Sisters of Charity of Saint Vincent De Paul) was founded eleven years later (1633) to serve the "poorest of the poor" and provide healthcare, followed in 1652 by the Sisters of Mercy of St. Borromeo with like charges, and many, many others.

In 1836 Theodor Fliedner, Lutheran Pastor of the poor municipality of Kaiserswerth (now part of Düsseldorf, Germany) formally reinstated the ministry of Deaconesses in and for the church. Inspired by the diaconate of the early Christian church and incorporating what he had seen on a visit to Mennonites in the Netherlands before, Fliedner set up an educational institution for Protestant Nurses where young, unmarried women received training in both theology and nursing skills according to a syllabus designed by him and his wife Friederike. The students lived in a house-church like environment observing daily prayers, Bible study, and the festival seasons of the church year. Fliedner's institution had an enormous impact throughout and beyond Europe. Florence Nightingale (1820–1910), one of the founders of modern nursing, visited Kaiserswerth in 1841 for the first time. She was so impressed by the devotion and practical expertise she experienced there that she returned to the place in 1850 for further training.

Learning Activities

- **Read**—Laboa's *"Helping the Sick"* (https://bit.ly/3OeN7RB).
- **Read**—Donahue's "Modern Nursing & the Nightingale Revolution" (https://bit.ly/3SoI3fT).

For Additional Reading

- **Read**—Murdarasi, "The Christian Faith of Florence Nightingale" (https://bit.ly/4289T3b), and Christian History Institute's "Healthcare and Hospitals in the Mission of the Church" (https://bit.ly/428Ls5G).
- **Reflect**—on the origin and meaning of *caritas*. What are ways to integrate *caritas* into your everyday life?

References

Benedict, N., Meisel, A., and del Mastro, M. (1975). *The Rule of St. Benedict*. Dumbarten Oaks Medieval Library Series. Crown Publishing Group.

Christian History Institute. (2011). *Christian History: Healthcare and Hospitals in the Mission of the Church*. 101. Worcester, PA. https://christianhistoryinstitute.org/uploaded/50cf8e35c4ae27.43897050.pdf.

Donahue, M. P. (1996). *Nursing, the Finest Art: Master Prints*. St. Louis / Baltimore / Boston: C.V. Mosby Co.

Ferngren, G. (2014). *Medicine and Religion: A Historical Introduction*. Johns Hopkins University Press.

Grundmann, C. H. (2018). "Christ as Physician: The Ancient *Christus medicus* Trope and Christian Medical Missions as Imitation of Christ." *Christian Journal for Global Health* 5, no. 3: 3–11. https://doi.org/10.15566/cjgh.v5i3.236.

Laboa, J. M. (2014). *Caritas: The Illustrated History of Christian Charity*. New York / Mahwah, NJ: Paulist Press.

Murdarasi, K. "The Christian Faith of Florence Nightingale: The Founder of Modern Nursing." *Premier Christianity* 11 May 2020. https://www.premierchristianity.com/home/the-christian-faith-of-florence-nightingale-the-founder-of-modern-nursing/2827.article.

Numbers, D., and Amundsen, D. (1986). *Caring and Curing: Health and Medicine in the Western Religious Traditions*. New York / London: Macmillan.

Reflection Questions for Group Discussion

1. What do you think was the purpose/meaning behind Jesus's healings?

2. Why did Jesus commission his disciples to heal and in which way does this impact the Christian healing ministry today?

3. How was the healing ministry carried out in the life of the early church?

4. How did Christians organize healthcare in the Middle Ages?

5. How did the reinstitution of the office of Deaconesses in the nineteenth century impact the development of professional nursing?

Lesson 5
Christian Medical Missions during the 19th and 20th Centuries

Summary	Knowledge Objectives
With the advent of modern rational-scientific medicine in the mid-nineteenth century it became possible to successfully treat diseases which until then decimated entire populations and caused unimaginable suffering on a grand scale. Pious physicians empowered by the gift of modern medicine perceived this as a call to action. They went out to share this gift with all who had no access to such help or lacked the means of obtaining it, irrespective if they lived nearby or far away. Thus, Christian medical missionaries became heralds of health around the globe taking medical care of people in need long before the establishment of the World Health Organization (WHO) and/or national ministries/departments of health. Christian medical missionaries also campaigned for proper sanitation to eradicate epidemics, set up medical and nursing schools, and challenged cultural practices wherever these stood in opposition to the Word of God.	1. Describe the emergence and development of medical missions in the mid-nineteenth century. 2. Name motivations and methods of Christian medical missions' pioneers. 3. Identify relevant reasons for the success and impact of Christian medical missions.
Thematic Content	**Attitude Objectives**
• Emergence of Christian medical missions in China in 1838 • Medical, pharmacological, and hygienic discoveries from 1846 to about 1950 • The global spread of Christian medical missions • Means of medical missions' work: hospitals, dispensaries, and itineration • The contribution of Christian medical missions to: 　» medical and nursing education 　» to women's liberation 　» to care for infants and children across cultures worldwide	1. Understand the connection between medical knowledge and the urge to make its benefits accessible for people in need wherever they are. 2. Verbalize awareness of the responsibility of being sent to heal. 3. Acknowledge the human tendency to pride and self-promotion and share what motivates you to consider the service of Christian healthcare.
Conceptual Thread—Healthcare and Healing	**Practice (Skills) Objectives**
The art of healing is as old as humankind. Since time immemorial people all over the world suffered from diseases and the effects of accidents. They, consequently, developed ways of treating various ailments. Without healing life cannot not be sustained as is obvious in the constant DNA repair. Healing is an expression of God's ongoing creation. That is why it was so important in the ministry of Jesus, and why it stays part of the eschatological hope of Christians, who believe that, finally, "death … mourning and crying and pain will be no more" (Rev 22:4). Healthcare workers are partakers in this godly ministry. They are called in a very specific way to witness to the corporeality of salvation in Christ.	1. Identify the aspects in biographies or autobiographies of global Christian healthcare workers/medical missionaries past or present that most appeal to you and explain why. 2. Explain the basic rationale behind the early heralds of health, their vision, and their commitment. 3. Describe the scope of Christian medical mission work when it reached its peak around 1930.

Part 1—The Emergence of Global Christian Medical Missions and Healthcare

Compassionate care for the sick, for lepers, and the needy of any sort was the hallmark of Christian responses to suffering for almost two millennia. But as the scientific age of medicine developed in the nineteenth century, the increasing ability to alter disease outcomes by physicians, proper medication and nursing became important components of Christian care. The importance of this step becomes clear when considering the medieval adage *Ubi tres medici, due athei* (Where three physicians [gather you'll find] two atheists [among them]). This primarily alluded to the pagan authorities of the medical profession (Hippocrates [460–377 BCE] and Galen [129–199 CE]), the abhorrence of magic, and later to the devout followers of René Descartes (1596–1650) who perceived the human being as a machine devoid of a soul.

The church, therefore, was initially quite suspicious of medicines and medical professionals, a suspicion that was not overcome until the mid-nineteenth century. Two reasons account for this change: first, the experiences of medically trained people in overseas mission fields, and second, the radical changes in the art of healing by applying the rational-scientific approach to medical practice leading to previously unimaginable advances in treatment and therapeutics.

Part 2—The Emergence of Medical Missions in Canton, China, in the 1830s

The concept of medical missions was not a brainchild of missionary strategists in Europe or the United States. It, rather, developed during the nineteenth century in the Far East, in Canton (now Guangzhu), China, in the context of commercial and religious enterprises. Only at Canton and only for a limited time each year were foreign merchants then permitted to trade with the otherwise secluded Chinese Empire at the so-called "Canton Factories." During these trading seasons physicians from Britain and the US responsible for the healthcare of the expatriate staff and the ships' crews also took residence there, as did some clerics. Contact with locals was strictly forbidden; foreigners were even prevented from learning Chinese.

Despite these restrictions Western physicians were approached by local people suffering from diseases for which there was no indigenous remedy, for example entropion, a widespread endemic disease of the eye where a lid folds inward making the lashes irritate and then damage the cornea causing severe inflammation and potential blindness. To correct it requires only a small surgical operation, which the Western-trained physicians could perform easily. Their Chinese colleagues lacked this skill, because surgery was not part of Chinese medicine at that time. Thus, a few philanthropically minded physicians, some of them Christians, responded to the need they found themselves confronted with by offering their services in temporary clinics whenever they were around, and their time permitted.

Part 3—Peter Parker and the Medical Missionary Society in China

Yale graduate Rev Peter Parker MD (1804–1888) entered this milieu as a missionary sent by the Boston-based American Board of Commissioners for Foreign Missions (ABCFM) in 1834. Qualified in both theology and medicine (with a brief special training in ophthalmology), and ordained a Presbyterian minister, Parker opened an Ophthalmic Hospital at Canton in 1835, which he dubbed P'u Ai I Yuan, Hospital of Universal Love. Originally intended as a place for treating eye diseases only, Parker soon had to attend to other illnesses as well. He even had to perform major surgeries when being asked to remove tumors, all of which, fortunately, turned out successfully (it was still a time without anesthesia and antisepsis!).

It is no surprise then that suffering Chinese, seeking healing of various ailments soon crowded his place, boldly ignoring the official prohibition of contact with foreigners. This brought the power of skilled medical work, especially surgery, to the attention of missionary strategists who eventually deemed medical work a convenient and legitimate means for establishing first contacts with people not otherwise accessible. Through the next decades medical missions became so important for mission strategy that in 1900 the influential British mission leader Herbert Lankester could speak of medical missions as "the heavy artillery of the missionary army" (*Students and the Missionary Problem*, London 1900, 494).

But the case for *medical* missions was not just hailed by people interested in mission. The Canton foreign business community, too, valued the enterprise. Its philanthropic character appealed to them as a convenient means for breaking down suspicion and prejudice of the "Foreign Devils" (*Fan-qui*) as the non-Chinese were called then. Such favorable assessment of Parker's hospital work proved critical since Parker was dependent on outside financial support because he offered his services in the spirit of genuine *disinterested benevolence* (see Box 2 below) free of charge. When Parker and his fellow missionaries failed to organize and institutionalize their benevolent medical work for the Chinese in 1836 due to insufficient funding from the Christian faith community in Europe and America, they turned to the businesspeople at Canton—Christian and non-Christian alike—who were more than willing to help. Missionaries and businessmen together founded the Medical Missionary Society in China in February 1838, the first of its kind ever. This Society was charged with the duty (1) to acquire qualified Christian physicians to staff the institutions at Canton and Macao (West of Canton), and (2) to collect contributions for running and maintaining these hospitals.

Learning Activities

- **Read**—"Disinterested Benevolence" (Box 2).
- **Read**—Grundmann's "The Medical Missionary Society in China" (https://bit.ly/3OAQ4fJ).
- **Reflect**—on the meaning of "Disinterested Benevolence." How do you demonstrate disinterested benevolence in your life and practice?

BOX 2 Disinterested Benevolence

In the first document soliciting support for medical missions published in 1836, Peter Parker and his colleagues at Canton wrote: "In order to attain the success of the object contemplated, those who engage in it must not receive any pecuniary *remuneration*: the work throughout must be, and appear to be, one of *disinterested benevolence*." (Original emphasis)

In his formative years Parker was exposed to and internalized a peculiar kind of serious personal piety—a piety inspired by the theological writings of Samuel Hopkins (1721–1803) who had transformed Jonathan Edwards' (1703–1758) theology into what may properly be called "evangelical Calvinism" which culminated in the concept of disinterested benevolence regarded as the hallmark of redeemed Christians. Its prototype was found in God offering his Son—and as such, offering himself on the cross for the redemption of all. Hopkins wrote:

> The highest instance of the most disinterested benevolence is ... that in which the divine character, or God's holy love, is acted out and set forth to our view. It hence appears that disinterested benevolence is the love in which God's holiness consists. Therefore, we are called upon to imitate this love of God, as that by which we may be like him, partakers of his holiness. ... If we love one another with that love which God exercised and manifested in giving his Son to die for us, we by this are conformed to God, his image is in us, and his love, which is his holiness, is complete and perfect in us. ... [T]he holiness of men consists in imitating this benevolent love. ("An Inquiry into the Nature of true Holiness" [1773], in *The Works of Samuel Hopkins*, Boston 1852, vol. III, 40f.)

Charles L. Chaney in his book *The Birth of Mission in America* (Pasadena, CA: William Carey Library 1976, 82f) writes:

> In the concept of disinterested benevolence the two great missionary motives, the glory of God and the salvation of man, became one. ... Disinterested benevolence provided a great impetus in the missionary movement for improving mankind's physical and social conditions. It also thereby became the primary defense for the missionary enterprise. ... Hopkins' peculiar eschatological slant helped to foster and direct this concern and to fashion the missionary character of the American churches as one concerned both with changing religious commitment and transforming human conditions. ... Disinterested benevolence, pregnant with social implications and concern, ... gave birth to a passion to minister to the physical needs of people. It fashioned the missionary thrust of the American churches not only into a bearer of culture but also into an agent of mercy.

Part 4—Scientific Medicine and Christian Medical Missions

The second reason for integrating professional medical work into Christian missions had to do with pivotal changes in the art of healing taking place during the second half of the nineteenth century when medicine turned from being an "art" into becoming a science. Epoch-making discoveries in medicine, surgery, hygiene, and pharmacology turned the classical healing art based on the study of ancient medical texts and personal experience, into evidence-based, rational-scientific medicine. To mention only a few of these discoveries: anesthesia and asepsis/antisepsis, both indispensable for safe surgery, were discovered as late as 1846/47. The importance of hygiene and proper sanitation, the basic requirements for public health and the prevention of many epidemics, were first realized during 1854–1859. In the 1850s and '60s cellular pathology and bacteriology became the cornerstones for diagnosis of diseases and the development of effective drugs and treatments.

Thus, in less than half a century the spell of the worst epidemics—leprosy, malaria, typhoid fever, tuberculosis, cholera, diphtheria, plague, yellow fever—was fading. What since time immemorial was perceived as caused by black magic, evil spirits, or as punishment by the wrath of God, now, suddenly became treatable and many could even be healed. Medicine, thus, became powerful and physicians got very euphoric. James L. Maxwell, General Secretary of the Medical Missionary Association of London, UK, interpreted these developments in 1914 as "God's hand in medical missions" explaining:

> The great mission work to the world had begun, but it was progressing very slowly. It needed what the medical art in service to Christ could alone give ... Today the medical missionary has in his hands a marvelously increased knowledge of the pathology and treatment of a great variety of diseases ... This constantly increasing knowledge has made the position of the medical missionary one of singular value for the propagation of the gospel. (Maxwell 1914, 67–69)

Part 5—Pious Christian Doctors Feel Urged to Share the Blessings with the Needy

As soon as the power of rational-scientific medicine became obvious, some Christian physicians, unlike most of their professional colleagues, realized the implicit responsibility which came along with the power of rational-scientific medicine, namely, to share it with all suffering people near and far. Providing relief of the "suffering of the heathen in times of illness" became imperative for them. Anyone responding negatively to this claim, either because of indifference or by focusing solely on their spiritual wellbeing, would have the deaths of "Murdered Millions" on their consciences. George D. Dowkontt, author of a book from 1897 by that very title, explains:

> While people discuss and question regarding the future of the heathen, they would do well, yes, better, to interrogate concerning the future prospects of those who, having the gospel for their spiritual needs, and medical science for their physical ills, enjoy the blessings of the same, but fail to send or give them to their needy fellow creatures ... Thus, do they [the needy fellow creatures] perish by our neglect... . Who is responsible for these lives if not those who could help them, but do not? Surely such are the murderers of these millions. To merely talk piously and tell suffering people of a future state, while neglecting to relieve their present needs, when in our power to do so, must be nauseating both to God and man, ... Christ ... combined care for the whole being of man, body and soul. (Dowkontt 1897, 17–18)

Part 6—Medical Missions Becomes an Established Feature of Missions

The assertion of the Ecumenical Missionary Conference held in New York City, April 21–May 1, 1900, that "No mission can be considered fully equipped that has not its medical branch" (*Report of the Conference* II, New York 1900, 199) indicates the importance and popularity given it then, although not everywhere and by everyone. Of the 128 North American missionary societies in existence around the turn to the twentieth century, only 37 (29%) were involved in medical missions; of the 154 British societies of that time only 45 (29%) were, and of the 82 continental ones only 14 (17%), totaling 96 or just 26%, all Protestant.

While Catholic religious orders continued to care for the sick in the traditional way as charitable works of mercy, they did not pursue *medical* missions at that time at all, save an initiative by French Cardinal Lavigerie to train African medical catechists at Valletta, Malta, in 1881, which, unfortunately, was doomed to failure by 1896. Only after appropriate changes in Canon Law were made during the twentieth century allowing for religious men and women (that is, for those having taken monastic vows) to practice medicine, did an increase in medical activities by Roman Catholic missionaries and religious orders become noticeable, particularly in the formation of the Society of Medical Missions Sisters (SMMS) in Washington, DC, in 1924, and the Medical Missionaries of Mary (MMM) in Ireland, in 1937.

Part 7—Means and Impact of Medical Missions

In the beginnings of medical missions, advances were often made through initiatives by highly motivated individuals setting up a small hospital at an accessible place as soon as they arrived at their designated location. These pioneers immediately co-opted and trained local assistants and began to do whatever they could under circumstances not favorable to the standards of hygiene to which they were accustomed.

But they toiled on, organizing dispensaries, and going on itineration visits to remote places in their area, distributing medicines and sharing the gospel. In the course of time, medical missionaries also began to establish professional organizations for doctors and nurses (the first of their kind in China and India). They also published scientific journals, translated medical reference works into Chinese and other languages, worked on an appropriate intercultural medical terminology (predating the *International Classification of Diseases*, ICD) and established medical and nursing schools for the training of indigenous personnel, some of these training institutions have become major medical schools in their country today (see Box 3 below).

Medical missionaries also offered careers in nursing and medicine for gifted people of the host countries and pioneered the inclusion of women into medical and nursing professions. Medical missionaries further opposed and actively campaigned against certain traditional customs affecting the health, even those like foot-binding in China and Sati (a widow's immolation on her husband's pyre) in India. They also opposed the custom of child marriages, opium consumption, and unhygienic sewage disposal. Female medical missionaries who had access to the women's quarters—Zenanas and Harems—in India, China, and Turkey (then the Ottoman Empire) contributed considerably to women's health (gynecology, obstetrics), the education and liberation of women, and the medical care of children (pediatrics) and their education. However, the work done in the hospitals—surgical procedures in particular—with a basic laboratory and a pharmacy well stocked with potent drugs remained preeminent in Christian medical missions throughout the late nineteenth and early twentieth centuries.

Learning Activities

- **Read**—"Overseas Christian Medical Colleges Then and Now" (Box 3 on next page).

- **Reflect**—What changes in doing medical missions have you noted in your reading? What were some of the early successes? Why did medical missionaries oppose and advocate against certain culturally accepted customs in countries like China, India, and the Ottoman Empire? Can you name some of these practices?

Christian Medical Missions during the 19th and 20th Centuries

BOX 3   Overseas Christian Medical Colleges Then and Now

1886—Founding of the Che Jung Wan Medical School (Medical School of Universal Helpfulness) in Seoul, Korea, by Dr. Horace N. Allen and Dr. J. W. Heron (Presbyterians from the US). In 1904 the school became the Severance Union Medical College (to honor the memory of one of its preeminent donors) and later the Yonsei University College of Medicine in Seoul, South Korea (http://medicine.yonsei.ac.kr/en/).

1894—Founding of the North Indian School of Medicine for Christian Women in Ludhiana, Punjab, as the first medical school for women in all of Asia by English Dr. (later, Dame) Edith Mary Brown sent by the Baptist Missionary Society, London. To comply with new government regulations and to admit male students too, in 1952 the institution became the Christian Medical College Ludhiana, a name by which it is still known today (http://www.cmcludhiana.in/).

1906—Founding of the Peking Union Medical College as a joint venture by various British and American mission societies. Handed over to the Rockefeller Foundation in 1915, which was eager to make it the Johns Hopkins of Asia. The college was nationalized in 1951 after the Marxist revolution and named China Union Medical College. Closed during the years of the Cultural Revolution in China (1966–1976) it was reopened in 1979 as Capital University of Medical Sciences before in 1985 it became Peking Union Medical College, again with the reputation of being one of the best in China. (https://www.pumch.cn/en.html).

1917—Founding of the Mengo Medical School at Kampala, Uganda, by Dr. (later, Sir) Albert Cook of the Church Missionary Society, London. In 2018 it became the Uganda Christian University School of Medicine (https://mengohospital.org/ucu-medical-school/).

1918—Founding of the Union Mission Medical School for Women in Vellore, Tamil Nadu, India, by Indian born American Dr. Ida Scudder of the Dutch Reformed Church in the United States of America. In 1938 the school was upgraded to a medical college, called the Christian Medical College, Vellore. Today it is one of the best medical colleges and hospitals in all of India (https://www.cmch-vellore.edu/).

Learning Activities

- **Read**—Grundmann's "Sent to Heal!: About the Biblical Roots, the History, and the Legacy of Medical Missions" (https://bit.ly/47Jx1X5).
- **Reflect**—What did the author share that resonated with you? What is the scope of your own missionary work?

References

Browne, S. G., Davey, F., and Porritt, L. (1985). *Heralds of Health: The Saga of Christian Medical Initiatives*. London: The Christian Medical Fellowship.

Dowkontt, G. (1897, reprint 2018). *Murdered Millions*. New York, NY: Forgotten Books.

Ecumenical Conference on Foreign Missions (1900). *Archival Collections*. Columbia, NY: University Libraries.

Grundmann, C. H. (2005). *Sent to Heal! Emergence and Development of Medical Missions*. Lanham, MD: University Press of America.

Grundmann, C. H. (2014). "Sent to Heal! About the Biblical Roots, the History, and the Legacy of Medical Missions." *Christian Journal for Global Health* 1, no. 1: 6–15. https://doi.org/10.15566/cjgh.v1i1.16.

Gulick, E. V. (1973). *Peter Parker and the Opening of China*. Cambridge, MA: Harvard University Press.

Wilkinson, J. (1990). *Making Men Whole: The Theology of Medical Missions*. London: The Christian Medical Fellowship.

Reflection Questions for Group Discussion

1. How did modern medical missions come about; where, when, and why?

2. What were arguments advanced for the cause of medical missions?

3. Why did Christian medical missions focus on hospitals and dispensaries?

4. What and in which way did Christian medical missions contribute to professional medical and nursing training around the world?

5. In which way did Christian medical missions contribute globally to women's health, their education, and liberation and to the healthcare of children?

Lesson 6
Christian Global Healthcare from the 20th to 21st Century

Summary	Knowledge Objectives
With the establishment of the WHO in 1947/48 and the formation of national ministries and departments of health, the overall situation of Christian medical missions changed considerably. Where the care of sick people by rational-scientific medical means once was completely shouldered by Christian hospitals, doctors, and nurses the work now became regulated by healthcare policies set and funded by secular governments overriding Christian priorities. Later, private hospitals and healthcare providers appeared, too, creating a competitive environment. This demanded a rethinking of the principles of Christian medical missions resulting in reorienting the focus from hospital centered care towards community health concerns by advocating Primary Health Care (PHC), a concept developed in the 1970s by the Christian Medical Commission (CMC) in cooperation with the WHO. Global Christian healthcare today is marked by providing basic healthcare for communities besides attentively listening to the needs of the people, mobilizing local resources to facilitate solutions from within the communities, and by committed cooperation as members of the body of Christ.	1. Describe the situation Christian medical missions faced after the end of World War II. 2. Explain the role CMC played in developing PHC. 3. Name reasons why medical missions morphed into healthcare missions and nowadays shows concern for the wider issues of justice and community-building (*shalom*), too.
Thematic Content	**Attitude Objectives**
• The emergence of global healthcare around the mid-twentieth century • Rethinking medical missions and the Tübingen Consultation of 1964 • The Primary Healthcare (PHC) approach • The new agenda for Christian medical missions • Christian medical missionaries once and now	1. Understand why the shift from hospital-centered care to community-based primary healthcare was deemed appropriate for Christian medical missions. 2. Devise means how genuine community participation in PHC programs can best be achieved. 3. Explain why Christian healthcare missions today require patient listening, committed cooperation, and genuinely being with the people.
Conceptual Thread—Corporeality of Salvation	**Practice (Skills) Objectives**
Global Christian healthcare represents a unique, yet vital ministry of the church. Healthcare workers are partakers in God's ongoing creative activity when bringing about healing through their medical expertise and nursing skill. They thereby witness to the corporeality of salvation in Christ. In so doing they safeguard the proclamation of the gospel from becoming a disembodied mental exercise and protect medical practice from turning into an exploitive materialistic undertaking. Thanks to such work medicine can stay truly humane and missions are prevented from falling prey to disembodied speculations and ideologies.	1. Acquire information about successful PHC projects run by local churches and/or Christian organizations. 2. Explain the need for community-based healthcare in contemporary Christian mission initiatives. 3. Discern how to respond to and set priorities for health-promoting missions in a community struggling with endemic diseases and other pressing healthcare needs in addition to facing economic disparities and educational deficiencies.

Part 1—Medical Missions in the 20th Century

The establishment of the World Health Organization (WHO) in 1947/48 promoted the worldwide creation of national healthcare services and Departments of Health. With the advent of national health services in the post-World War II period and the emancipation of colonies from foreign governments, the overall environment of medical missions changed considerably. Medical missionaries and their sending organizations were now required to comply with WHO standards and national healthcare policies and had to cooperate with colleagues not interested in sharing the gospel. In most cases such cooperation did not present serious issues, at least not initially, because in their nascent state the emerging national healthcare administrations were heavily dependent on existing infrastructures and examples maintained by Christian medical missions regarding institutions, personnel, training, and finances.

However, in the latter half of the twentieth century, estrangement set in. In China and some African and South Asian regions, church-owned healthcare facilities were nationalized, and Christian distinctiveness eradicated (as in China) and/or minimized. In most sub-Saharan African countries and in India ownership of institutions and programs was transferred to local churches, which now operated in parallel with growing government-sponsored services, but without any of the public subsidy nearby district hospitals received. Later still, other healthcare facilities were built, national as well as private ones, some for-profit, but some also not-for-profit. National experts had now the final word in every respect.

While they had blazed the trail to bring healing to the poor and suffering to even the remotest of regions as "heralds of health," Christian medical missions now stood in competition with other similar enterprises increasingly better staffed and effectively managed. Government institutions were now tasked with the responsibility to provide healthcare for all citizens of a given region and nation, at least in theory. What was the role of Christian mission hospitals in this context? Should church hospitals and clinics stay in this kind of competition? Should Christian healthcare workers carry on or should funds for the upkeep of medical institutions and the salary of medical personnel be diverted to other non-health-related missionary projects regarded as more central to the task of mission? How could Christian healthcare missions and the people engaged therein remain true to the Christian calling?

Learning Activities

- **Read**—McGilvray's "The Beginning of the Christian Medical Commission" (https://bit.ly/3HsHqM3).
- **Read**—McGilvray's "The World Health Organization and Primary Health Care" (https://bit.ly/3SuonHM).
- **Read**—Hilton's "The Future of Medical Missions" (https://bit.ly/47Fjq32).
- **Reflect**—Upon creative ways to make healthcare services become more meaningful to communities at large.

Part 2—Rethinking Medical Missions

To address the uncertainties of the future state of Christian medical missions aired by many in the field, a conference was convened at Tübingen, Germany, late in May 1964 organized by the World Council of Churches (WCC) together with the Lutheran World Federation (LWF). Since many of their member bodies had huge stakes in medical missions, they had a serious interest in coming to terms with the new challenges. Contrary to what participants expected beforehand, namely, to let go of medical work in missions, one of them reported afterwards, the "consultation discovered in a quite unplanned way that to ask whether or not the time has come for the church to surrender its work in medicine … is to ask a *theological* question." Before Tübingen, "Consultation participants leaned in the direction of the church withdrawing from areas of healing now strongly occupied by the state." But "the Consultation was led to articulate the belief that 'the Christian church has a specific task in the field of healing.'" (WCC 1964, 470–71).

To the surprise of all, the "Findings" of the conference got enthusiastic approval by those actively engaged in medical missions worldwide. It helped them redefine their identity as genuinely partaking in a vital Christian agency, namely in the healing ministry of the church. The Tübingen conference also led to the formation of the WCC's Christian Medical Commission (CMC) in 1968 as the global advocate of medical mission concerns and the Christian counterpart to the WHO. Its mandate was to "promote … joint planning and action (a) between … churches … and (b) between … other voluntary agencies and the Government," but also to "undertake and encourage the study of the nature of the Christian ministry of healing and the problems which confront it [i.e., the healing ministry] in a changing world (McGilvray 1981, 42).

The CMC conducted several consultations and studies on the healing ministry of the church in various places around the world and helped establish worldwide networking and cooperation among Christian healthcare programs including those run by the Roman Catholic Church. The CMC also dialogued with the WHO and backed by results from the study process, became instrumental in developing the Primary Health Care approach (PHC). After analyzing the contribution hospital care made to the overall state of health of entire populations, it turned out that the impact of such institutional care was far less than expected yet required the lion's share of the budget, namely 80 percent.

To become more effective, it was determined that funds should be directed with a focus on the local people and their health concerns first. These concerns included, among others, prevention, and treatment of common diseases by providing sanitation, sufficient and nutritious food, safe drinking water, mother-and-child care, supplying basic drugs and vaccines, and engaging in health education and outreach programs. Instead of placing hospitals everywhere, the PHC approach promoted a tiered referral system starting with a basic and very simple village health-post managed by local healthcare workers and supported by secondary or even tertiary care medical facilities, that is general and specialized hospitals staffed with qualified medical experts. This approach became the declared official WHO policy in 1978 by its General Assembly meeting in Alma Ata, USSR (now, Almaty, Kazakhstan) and was emphatically reaffirmed thirty years later in "*The World Health Report 2008: Primary Health Care Now More Than Ever*" (WHO, Geneva, Switzerland, 2008).

Bidding farewell to heroic medical initiatives by highly motivated individuals and deemphasizing the once so prestigious, publicly noticeable institutions like hospitals and dispensaries was not easy. Yet, the transition towards primary health care was felt necessary for staying faithful to the healing mission of the church. Consequently, Christian medical missions began shifting the focus to training of local people, to community-based healthcare work, to cooperation in partnerships, and the enablement of local healthcare initiatives. The emphasis on hospital care gave way in many cases to a more preventative approach with a focus on the health of communities at large. What was formerly known as *medical missions* was transitioning (or maturing), thus, into more broadly conceptualized *healthcare missions* addressing also issues of justice and healthy community-building. This approach proved its efficiency by having an unprecedented positive impact on the actual well-being of entire populations. It led to innovative healthcare projects, many of which were/are conceived of and run by local Christians, who also often assumed responsibility for the work in former mission hospitals. Only a small sample of such projects and associations is given below (Box 4).

The following is a small sample of associations of professional cooperation among former mission hospitals and comprehensive healthcare projects managed by local Christians (the list has been arranged chronologically).

BOX 4   Overseas Christian Medical Colleges Then and Now

1 Christian Medical Association of India (CMAI)

"In 1905, a group of missionary doctors set up the Medical Missionary Association of India to provide Christian medical professionals with a forum for sharing and supporting each other spiritually and professionally. The organization was renamed Christian Medical Association of India in 1926. … We work through the church, CMAI's network of members and the government." (https://www.cmai.org/who-we-are/about-cmai.html)

2 Catholic Health Association of India (CHAI)

"From its humble beginnings in … 1943, the Catholic Health Association of India has grown into the world's largest health care organization in the voluntary sector." (https://chai-india.org/)

3 Emmanuel Hospital Association in India: URL

"The origins of EHA can be found in the late 1960s when a group of Indian and international leaders and health care workers met together to look for appropriate ways to bring about long-term sustainability of some 13 former mission hospitals … The twenty years between 1950 and 1970 were the "dark ages" of medical missions in India. In the 1950's hundreds of European missionaries began to leave India. This sudden and large-scale exodus left many medical missions and churches in a crisis of leadership and funding. Mission hospitals … were finding it hard to recruit fresh personnel. Even when they did, restrictions on grant of visas to foreign missionaries posed serious problems. Mission institutions began to close. This had a huge impact on the health care of Indians, since in 1950 one in every three hospital beds in India was to be found in a mission hospital. … It was in such a milieu that the idea of a federation of mission hospitals came into being. It was in the year 1970 that EHA was officially formed. … Over the years EHA has grown to be a medical missionary movement and a fellowship of Christian health professionals committed to bring about wholeness of life to the marginalized members of our varied communities." (https://eha-health.org/)

4 Comprehensive Rural Health Project, Jamkhed, Maharashtra, India

Founded in 1970 by the Christian "Drs. Raj and Mabelle Arole to bring healthcare to the poorest of the poor, CRHP has become an organization that empowers people and communities to eliminate injustices through integrated efforts in health and development. CRHP works by mobilizing and building the capacity of communities to achieve access to comprehensive development and freedom from stigma, poverty, and disease. Pioneering a comprehensive approach to community-based primary healthcare (also known as the Jamkhed Model), CRHP has been a leader in public health and development in rural communities in India and around the world." (https://www.crhpindia.org/)

5 Evangelical Medical Fellowship of India (EMFI)

Founded in 1974 EMFI sees itself as a "Fellowship for promoting wholistic medical services among the poor, needy, and unreached in India in the name of Jesus Christ" desiring to represent "Christ's transforming presence in healthcare and the nation through Christ-centered medical professionals." (https://emfi.in/)

6 Health for One Million (HOM)

Also founded in 1974, "HOM is a comprehensive health service wing of the Diocese of Marthandam," housed at St. John's Hospital in Trivandrum/ Thiruvananthapuram, Kerala, India. It aims "at the total development of the people" with women playing "the main role in HOM programmes. … The principles of Health for One Million are that "Health care is more important than disease cure; health can be maintained only in the context of total human development; development means self-growth; community development means community growth from within; self-help and self-sustained programmes are the most effective; community decision is more meaningful than community participation alone; formal as well as informal education methods are adopted to educate people on Health and development." In (http://healthforonemillion.com/)

7 Overseas Medical Mission Center, Changhua Christian Hospital, Taiwan (CCH)

In 1988 CCH began its overseas medical service, "with the core value of 'SHARE' which means Spirit, Health, Alliance, Resource and Education. … CCH overseas medical teams … covered Africa, Asia, [the] South Pacific and Caribbean regions which included Swaziland, Sao Tome and Principe, Papua New Guinea, Myanmar, Vietnam, Mongolia, Thailand, St. Vincent, and St. Lucia as well." CCH hosted "medical staffs and/or pastors from developing countries and designed short-term training courses based on their needs. … Medical personnel from Africa, South Pacific, Asia, and Caribbean regions [visit] CCH for one to three months training in the fields of hospital management, patient care, nursing care, medical laboratory, pediatrics, biomedical engineering etc." (https://www2.cch.org.tw/cch_english)

8 Pan African Academy of Christian Surgeons (PAACS)

PAACS emerged from a partnership with Loma Linda University and the Christian Medical and Dental Association (CMDA) as "a non-denominational Christian organization in 2003 for the training of general surgeons in Africa called 'Pan-African College of Christian Surgeons'. In 2004 the name was changed to 'Pan-African Academy of Christian Surgeons'" which became an independent ministry in 2020, "serving the Lord as a stand-alone organization, training and mentoring African physicians as surgeons to care for the poor and share the love of Christ with those in need." (https://paacs.net/)

9 Africa Christian Health Associations Platform (ACHAP)

"An advocacy and networking platform for Christian Health Associations (CHAs) and Church Health Networks from Sub-Saharan Africa" established through "the inspiration and support of the World Council of Churches in 2007." Legally registered as a Non-Governmental-Organization (NGO) in Nairobi, Kenya, in 2012, ACHAP promotes "continued, effective and efficient engagement of Church Health Services in Africa towards achieving equitable access to quality health care among members of the Platform and in Africa at large. … and partners in support of the Church health work in Africa." (https://africachap.org/)

Part 3—Christian Global Healthcare Missions in the 21st Century

The overall conditions for Christian global healthcare missions have changed significantly since the nineteenth century. Today it is no longer possible to go elsewhere simply with the intention of doing good by providing healthcare for suffering people. As laudable as the desire to help is, it is shortsighted when done without proper consideration, thoughtful reflection, and cultural preparation beforehand (see Lessons 7–9). Actionist do-gooding often turns out counterproductive and, thus, may jeopardize the gospel witness.

Aspiring candidates for global Christian healthcare missions will be faced with a host of obstacles, beginning with obtaining a working permit, being willing to cooperate with non-Christian colleagues, working under superiors not always professionally as competent as desired, and coping with shortages of means and strange working environments. These stresses are compounded by challenges posed by language barriers and cultural chasms while caring for the long queue of sick individuals who arrive for medical care, but also by engaging in prevention and attending to health issues of the wider community like suffering from injustice or social oppression.

These difficulties cannot be done away with simply by pointing to good intentions like freely offering time and expertise or bringing medications and funds along. Good intentions are good, but not good enough for this ministry. Such ministry demands more. For the success of the enterprise, it is of utmost importance that every aspiring Christian global healthcare mission worker *listens* first—and long (1) to discern if there is a genuine personal call for such work and (2) to truly understand the people and population one wants to help, their way of life and their way of coping with the challenges life presents—so as to be able to make an honest assessment one's own role and working context. Only then will it be possible to begin the journey to become a means of healing for the people group one wants to serve. Disinterested benevolence for Christ's sake will be demonstrated best by really listening to the needs of the local people, addressing their actual concerns and healthcare issues, assessing the human resources and material means present, and then, collaboratively devising a plan of action based on medical and nursing expertise of how best to achieve the set goals. All of this requires professional competence that invites input by all qualified persons, irrespective of religious affiliation.

This implies also setting aside selfish interests and vested obligations for the sake of a clear focus on how best to relieve the sufferers of their ailments. What counts is professional and spiritual competence, not compliance with a hidden agenda or self-aggrandizement. However, while being competent, listening, collaborating, and giving compassionate care that is different, Christians are not silent about the "hope that is within," which motivates them to engage in such ministry in the first place. Christians are winsome all the time by means of listening dialogue and distinct lifestyles that may bring a person to awareness of the Healer behind all that is being done.

Christian healthcare workers thereby imitate Christ who emptied himself to become the servant of all (Phil 2:5–8). Imitating Christ this way will prompt questions as to the "why" and "how" of selfless giving. People will also notice the affiliation with the Christian community, the observing of times of prayer and worship, the study of the Bible, and the general conduct of life. Christian global health ministry goes far beyond the mere professional and economic exchange. It becomes a way of life and a profound witness.

Learning Activities

- **Read**—Downing's "Global Health Means Listening" (https://bit.ly/47Fjq32).

- **Reflect**—Why is listening so important when caring for others?

Part 4—Cooperation with Non-Christians

One hindrance of advancing global Christian healthcare work today is the necessity to cooperate with people who do not share the Christian faith. This applies to many workplaces at home. But this aspect requires special attention in the case of global Christian healthcare missions as to how such projects explicitly can bear witness to the corporeality of salvation in Christ in the context of different religious and cultural settings.

With national healthcare systems in place nowadays and qualified medical staff often (but not always) locally available, those stepping from outside into a different culture come as foreigners and strangers. Yet, they must comply with the rules and regulations of the accreditation and licensing councils of their host country and abide by the legal and reporting procedures of its Ministry of Health and its other agencies. Working within the jurisdiction of local Ministry of Health authorities, who sometimes have little experience or questionable qualifications, expatriate healthcare workers may experience resistance to their good intentions and sometimes feel at odds with the system in place—even when on short-term emergency relief or development missions. Whether coming alongside to work in a church health system, a Ministry of Health facility, or a secular non-governmental organization, the frame of action is set by the host country's Ministry of Health's understanding of being responsible for the health of its citizens. This requires due recognition and collaboration.

Learning Activities

- **Read**—"Corporeality of Salvation" (Box 5, below).
- **Reflect**—What does it mean that God became incarnate in Jesus Christ, and how does that inform what you do as part of the body of Christ?

BOX 5   Corporeality of Salvation

"The body is the pivot of salvation." This pointed statement was made in the third century AD in the treatise "On the resurrection of the flesh/the body" by Tertullian (ca. 160–220), a Father of the Church from North Africa. Tertullian alerts to creation, the incarnation, and to the bodily resurrection to show that any merely "spiritual" gospel-talk is missing the essential. The incarnation, Tertullian explains, happened precisely for the sake of sustaining and redeeming humans with their frail body (not: redeeming them from their body!) as Jesus's ministry illustrates, especially his healings.

To assume that humans are composites of "body," "soul," and "mind" or to perceive persons as "ensouled bodies" has become the common anthropological paradigm today. However, the mind-body/body-soul dichotomy is a Neoplatonic (3rd–6th century) legacy, not a biblical one. Terminological constructs like "holistic" or "wholistic" try to compensate for some of the noticed deficiencies of this concept, but unlike the phrase "corporeality of salvation," they fail to overcome the mind-body/body-soul dualisms.

The corporeality of salvation emphasizes the biblical view of God's redemptive act in Jesus Christ over against modernistic concepts which tend to compartmentalize the claim of the gospel according to preconceived theories of nature or the human being as expressed in the body-mind dichotomy. The biblical view is comprehensive. It acknowledges that nothing is bodiless; even the most abstract of ideas is dependent on a comprehending brain. God created the world, that is the broad variety of living beings past and present in all forms of appearance.

God became incarnate in Jesus Christ, who healed everyone seeking his help and who was concerned about the wellbeing of humans (John 10:10), so much so, that he counted care for the needy, whoever they were, as decisive for the ruling in the last judgment (Matt 25:31–46). Resurrection is also conceived biblically as a corporeal event (1 Cor 15:35–56), because personal identity hinges on bodily existence. We don't have a body, we are body!

Part 5—Commitment and Short-Term Healthcare Missions

The history of Christian medical missions reveals that one of the most important virtues of its agents was genuine commitment. Medical missionaries and healthcare workers did not mind obstacles or threats to their health or to their own lives (as was the case in China during the Boxer rebellion, 1899–1901). Many authenticated their calling by toiling on, turning stumbling blocks into steppingstones while some also endured the ultimate sacrifice. Today, however, global Christian healthcare missions face new possibilities which might impinge upon that very virtue. The convenience of air-travel as well as high-speed global communication now have made short-term medical mission trips a common feature of global Christian healthcare ministries. Such ventures make perfect sense in situations where experts make themselves available for treating clearly defined diseases like cleft lips or cataracts in well prepared camps for a select triaged patient population.

Short-term medical missions may also play a part in emergency relief after earthquakes, flooding, hurricanes, famine, and war, provided they do not stay independent but work in cooperation with the authorities in place. Another meaningful short-term assignment consists in briefly filling in for unforeseen staffing shortages in hospitals or healthcare projects as a sign of worldwide Christian solidarity or participating in training of local healthcare personnel to build healthcare capacity. However, when sending students on short-term missions or for service-learning experiences, the case looks somewhat different. Such exposures are marvelous educational means for their benefit. In experiencing the differences of language, culture, religions, and people, the students, hopefully, come to realize the peculiarity of their own culture and background and their personal inclinations. Yet, their actual contribution to the healthcare projects may be minimal.

Global Christian healthcare missions require authentic commitment by everyone involved in it, a commitment not reducible to spectacular short-term actions. Christian healthcare missions are to be reliable, sustainable, and sacrificial so that their beneficiaries do not get humiliated as mere recipients of charitable crumbs falling from the table of those who have plenty. Only when such an attitude gets embraced wholeheartedly will those who benefit from healthcare intervention from outside be enabled to become transformative agents of health themselves.

Learning Activities

- **Read**—Crespo's "Community Health: From Delivery to Responsibility" (https://bit.ly/42b0ecm).
- **Read**—Ewert's "Trends in Medical Missions" (https://bit.ly/42bVYsU).
- **Reflect**—What responsibilities should global Christian healthcare workers keep in mind when serving others and promoting community health?

Part 6—Seeking the Opportunity: The Message of Global Christian Healthcare Missions

Christian medical missions once were the first of their kind in many places. But in today's world, medical missions are also carried out by other non-faith-based organizations. It is no surprise, then, that many actively involved in medical missions thought that the time had come to pull out and hand over the work to secular civil authorities. However, the Tübingen consultation's "Findings" made them reconsider because medical services, too, are part of the healing ministry of the church, a ministry mandated by her Lord and Master (see Lesson 4). The church as "the corporate fellowship of the People of God wherever it manifests itself" (WCC 1964, 35) cannot surrender this ministry to other agencies.

The historical overview of Christian medical/health care missions teaches us important lessons:

- Efforts at healing are an integral part of the gospel. They emphasize the bodily, corporeal dimension of salvation, a dimension which undeniably was a feature of Jesus's ministry. The global church must—not exclusively, of course—avail of medical healing, not just for promoting health itself but as a sign of the life abundant which Jesus came to bring (John 10:10) and as a witness to God's ongoing creation. The church must also engage in medicine and provide for wholistic healthcare for medicine to stay truly humane. This is particularly true in our times with modern, rational-scientific medicine and its ever-expanding, technically-driven possibilities (like manipulating the genetic makeup of life yet unborn, and by prolonging a person's lifespan).

- The church's healing ministry must stay engaged globally because its understanding of health stretches beyond mere medical and healthcare concerns. It also includes proclamation of the gospel in the way medicine, nursing, or public health is practiced across cultures. The good news of the gospel is also good news for medical practitioners, namely, to liberate them from the hubris to fight death by all means or to focus on diseases only. Christian healthcare personnel should be the first to recognize that medicine or public health is to prevent untimely death, but not death as such, since death cannot be overcome by medicine. The gospel message to be proclaimed to medicine and her practitioners is that death is overcome in Jesus Christ already once and for all (1 Cor 15:54–57). This enables all to become more realistic about what can be done, what should be done, and what to abstain from. Global Christian healthcare mission also renders another, unique service to medicine by keeping alive the awareness that to be concerned about healing implies being concerned also about the larger circumstances of the life of individual patients, namely their social, economic, religious, cultural, and political environment, and—as being created in the image of God—their entitlement to experience dignity and (*shalom*).

- Finally, global Christian healthcare missions are initiatives by all God's people, not just by the professionally trained, committed individuals or groups directly involved in it. The work done by physicians, nurses, public health workers, and ancillary staff in hospitals and health programs is dependent not only on backing by the larger Christian community for the provision of funds and administrative support. Such work is dependent also on the respective medical community becoming a lively part of actual church life in given congregations who pray with the people of God and are prayed for by the people of God. It is this all-comprehensive lived mutuality as a people of God which makes Christian healthcare ministries recognizable as such. That is and remains their distinctive feature.

Learning Activities

- **Read**—Kuhn, "Too Many Patients, Too Little Time: What Can I Do?" (https://bit.ly/4918Zb6).
- **Reflect**—How does one navigate healthcare as a Christian when there are too many patients but too little time?

References

Downing, R. (2018). *Global Health Means Listening*. Nairobi: Manqa Books.

Ewert, D. M. (1998). *A New Agenda for Medical Missions*. Brunswick, GA: MAP International.

Germany, C. (1964). "The Healing Ministry." *International Review of Missions* 53: 470–71.

Grundmann, C. H. (2005). *Sent to Heal! Emergence and Development of Medical Missions*. Lanham, MD: University Press of America.

Grundmann, C. H. (2015). "The Legacy of Tübingen I: On the Occasion of Its Fiftieth Anniversary." *International Review of Mission*, Geneva, Switzerland, WCC 104, no. 1: 118–33.

Kuhn, W. T. (2014). *Heal in Imitation of Christ: Conversations on Medical Missions*. Sisters, OR: Trusted Books.

Litsios, S. (2004). "The Christian Medical Commission and the Development of the World Health Organization's Primary Health Care Approach." *American Journal of Public Health* 94, no. 11: 1884–93.

McGilvray, J. (1981). *The Quest for Health and Wholeness*. Tübingen, German Institute for Medical Missions.

World Council of Churches—WCC (1964). Geneva, Switzerland.

World Health Organizations (2008). "The World Health Report 2008: Primary Health Care Now More Than Ever." Geneva, Switzerland.

Reflection Questions for Group Discussion

1. What is the legacy of the Tübingen conference of 1964?

2. What was the Christian input to the development of the Primary Health Care (PHC) approach of the WHO?

3. Why is it that Christian medical missions (or: Global Christian healthcare work) needed reconsideration in the middle of the twentieth century?

4. What does it mean to witness the corporeality of salvation in Christ when engaging in healthcare ministries?

5. How can global Christian healthcare missions be conducted in such a way that they witness to God's desire "that all may have life, and have it abundantly" (John 10:10)?

6. In which way are global Christian healthcare missions initiatives by all of God's people?

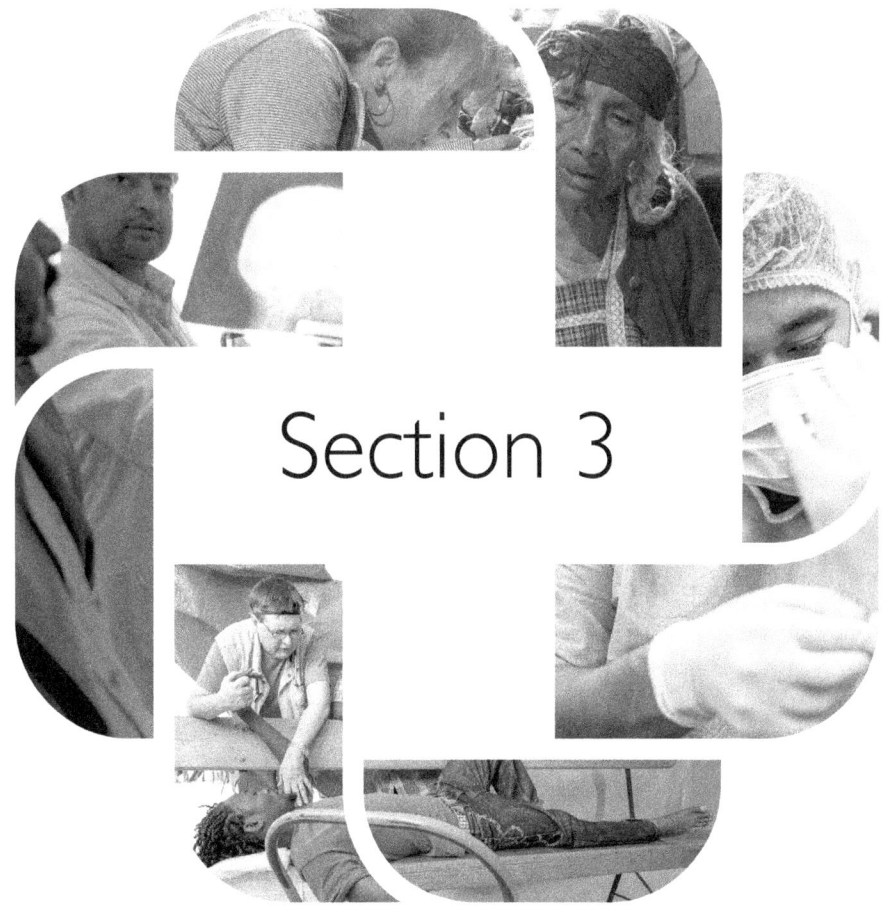

Section 3

Cultural Perspectives

Rebecca Meyer and Grace Tazelaar

Lesson 7
Worldview, Culture, and Health

Summary	Knowledge Objectives
Cultures around the world have differing worldviews, practices, and behaviors related to health, disease, healing, suffering, death, and dying. Healthcare and ministry workers need to learn how to integrate that understanding with a kingdom worldview. A kingdom worldview has been revealed in Scripture, is true, trustworthy, and guides believers. Creation, the fall, redemption, and restoration is one way of viewing God's kingdom. It begins with *shalom* and ends with *shalom*.	1. Discuss the concept of culture and its influence on worldview. 2. Compare major worldviews and ways to interact with people who have different worldviews to minimize cultural distress. 3. Evaluate the importance of a person's culture/worldview/religion on their healthcare decisions and the ways it shapes values, beliefs, morality, and behavior.
Thematic Content	**Attitude Objectives**
• Definition of terms and concepts related to culture. • How culture, worldview, and religion shape decisions made by people around the world. • Sample culture, worldviews, and religions and their perspective on healing and salvation.	1. Appreciate the effects of secular worldviews on current practices of health and healing. 2. Increase personal awareness of how different beliefs, values, religion, language, and other cultural factors influence health promotion.
Conceptual Thread—Culture	**Practice (Skills) Objectives**
Culture can be defined as the learned behaviors, values, beliefs, and faith or view of reality, that influence a person's definition of life, health, and illness. Culture may also include ethnicity, socioeconomic status, ability or disability, sexual orientation, age, and occupation or profession. **Conceptual Thread—Worldview** A worldview (or vision of life) is a framework or set of fundamental beliefs through which we view the world and our part in it. It is the deepest level of culture and affects every aspect of health, including the choices people make about suffering, death, and dying.	1. Give two examples of ways that worldview, beliefs, and values shape people's behavior and impacts their health. 2. Identify some of your own potential biases based on your worldview. 3. Identify a personal strategy to develop cross-cultural awareness and humility.

Part 1—Terms and Concepts

The next three lessons present a biblical, wholistic perspective about culture, worldview, and ways to serve in cross-cultural contexts while sharing the gospel with those who do not know the Lord. The writers of this content know that there is no way that all cultures, beliefs, and practices can be included in so short a document—so these lessons will provide a broad overview with the hope that the learner will dig deeper into areas of personal interest.

God has called his people to join him on mission, the *Missio Dei*, and all that he is doing in the world. The task is not just to make disciples and plant churches in all the geopolitical places of the world, but rather to reach, make disciples, baptize, and teach *panta ta ethne* (all the nations)—all the ethnolinguistic people groups of the world. The world as we know it is ever-changing which creates new challenges for reaching and teaching all peoples, including a growing number of people following Islam, changing global economies, new technologies, pandemics, devastating wars, displaced populations, environmental changes, and natural disasters. Navigating in this changing world is a challenge and there have been many discussions, literature, and research in the past few decades about the best way to serve in different ethnolinguistic groups or cultures. This lesson will present a few terms and concepts related to culture from a combined anthropology and missiology perspective to lay the foundation for the content (Pratt, Sills, and Walters, 2014).

Culture is a term that is used in many ways and in disciplines such as anthropology, psychology, medicine, public health, social work, and nursing, and it encompasses more than just ethnicity and nationality. It is the learned and shared beliefs, values, and patterns of behavior in any group of people that is passed on from generation to generation. Every people group around the world has its own rules for living, working, communicating, worshiping, their own heart language, and their own beliefs and values (Pratt, Sills, and Walters, 2014).

There is the visible aspect of culture that a person can see and hear, such as language, food, and clothes, and less visible components such as patterns of speech and behavior, family traditions, and roles of various family members. Culture also includes many other aspects of life, such as gender, age, physical abilities, religious affiliation, educational status, socioeconomic status, occupation, military experience, political beliefs, and urban versus rural residence. Every encounter with a person can be a cross-cultural encounter, even the person living next door.

Healthcare and ministry workers taking the gospel to the ends of the earth need to recognize that health and illness (or wellness) is shaped by a person's culture and their worldview. A biblical or kingdom worldview gives us all common language and understanding of God's purposes in disease, suffering, death, and healing. Culture, beliefs, values, and worldview influences everything that people choose to do and what they believe, so it is important to define these terms. Lesson 8 will focus more on culturally determined factors, such as individualism versus collectivism, circular versus linear thinking, fatalism, and locus of control.

Defining Culture

There are many definitions of the term culture, many of which converge on the view that culture is a social construct, or idea, which is not genetic or inherited. Culture includes the values, behavior, norms, beliefs, and worldview of persons, communities, and populations. According to Giger (2017), "it is a patterned behavioral response that develops over time as a result of imprinting the mind through social and religious structures and intellectual and artistic manifestations" (2).

Culture is also the product of the interaction between people and their environments. Culture consists of shared elements within that environment, and people can belong to many "cultures": ethnicity, religion, generation, sexuality, occupation, education, and socioeconomic status. Culture is transmitted from person to person across time and generations (Triandis 2007, as cited in Giger 2017). Cumulatively, "culture" is the set of characteristics and psychosocial environment in which the person is situated, and which informs how they navigate the world.

Culture implies a measure of homogeneity. But, if the unit is larger than the clan or small tribe, a culture will include within itself several subcultures, and subcultures of subcultures, within which a wide variety and diversity is possible. Jesus himself came into the Jewish culture, a subculture of a larger Ancient Near East culture, to serve others and accomplish the redemption of believers regardless of their cultural or ethnic background (Elmer 2006).

According to the Lausanne Willowbank Report (1978),

> At its center, culture is part of a worldview, that is, a general understanding of the nature of the universe and of one's place in it. This may be "religious" (concerning God, or gods and spirits, and of our relation to them), or it may express a "secular" concept of reality, as in a Marxist society. From this basic worldview flow both standards of judgement or values (of what is good in the sense of desirable, of what is acceptable as in accordance with the general will of the community, and of the contraries) and standards of conduct (concerning relations between individuals, between the sexes and the generations, with the community and with those outside the community). Culture is closely bound up with language, and is expressed in proverbs, myths, folk tales, music, and various art forms…It governs actions undertaken in community—acts of worship or of general welfare; laws and the administration of law; social activities such as dances and games; smaller units of action such as clubs and societies, associations for an immense variety of common purposes. (4–5)

Cultural Humility

The Willowbank Report also discusses the concepts of humility, respect, and servanthood. According to Scripture, humility is an attitude believers need to adopt, especially when working cross-culturally, "Clothe yourselves in humility" (1 Pet 5:5). The expression of humility may be culturally determined. However, when believers take the time to appreciate other cultures and beliefs, bridges will be built. When serving others, believers can show understanding, establish trust, build relationships, and be open to learning new things (Elmer 2006). Healthcare literature tends to use the term "cultural competence" when providers interact well with the diverse populations seen across the globe. However, the idea of cultural competence can imply superiority, where one person is labeled competent, and another is not. The preferred term, especially from a biblical perspective, is cultural humility.

Cultural humility is an ongoing process where healthcare workers and ministry partners self-reflect on their own beliefs and values while working hard to understand the culture, worldview, and cultural practices of others. According to Elmer, humility and a servant's heart is important: "Missionaries [and those working cross-culturally] could more effectively minister the gospel of Christ if they did not think they were so superior…" (2006, 15). Cultural awareness, that is, having an appreciation of diverse cultural groups and their language, lifestyle, arts, dress, music, and foods, provides a cross-cultural worker the ability to demonstrate cultural humility, genuine commitment, and the love of God. Being culturally sensitive is also important, which includes using sensitive language, being aware of what is going on regarding where people sit (status) who eats first, and the roles of each person, and not saying things or behaving in ways that may be seen as offensive to someone (communication).

Healthcare workers who have been educated to value and practice from a scientific worldview often have implicit cultural bias without even realizing they do, so it is important to be aware of this potential bias when caring for others. Implicit bias is having a certain attitude toward people or having associated stereotypes without being conscious of it. For example, when someone doesn't follow health advice or instructions, healthcare personnel may label that person as non-compliant before taking the time to learn that person's view of the health situation. Perhaps the person cannot afford the medication, or maybe they are not able to read the instructions. In her book, *The Spirit Catches You and You Fall Down*, Anne Fadiman repeatedly illustrates how healthcare personnel and a Hmong refugee family talk past one another, resulting in poor outcomes for the patient. Wholistic care did not occur in that situation.

Using cultural humility includes the ability to approach another person with openness, compassion, and the love of Jesus, without making stereotypical assumptions or judgments. When using this method to approach those being cared for, the healthcare worker and ministry partners assume a learning posture and not one of power and control. If living and serving overseas or in a different cultural context within your own neighborhood, one fundamental way to help develop this humble, servant mind-set is to learn the language, which will be discussed more in the next lesson (Yeager and Bauer-Wu 2014). The most important thing is to treat people with dignity and respect. Suffering affects people on all levels—body, mind, soul, and spirit. The ability to listen well, as has been discussed in previous lessons, confirm and acknowledge what has been seen without judgment allows the healthcare worker and ministry partners to share the struggle with the person who is suffering. Good dialogue establishes trust and a willingness to learn from the other person (Elmer 2006).

Learning Activities

- **Write** a brief definition of the following terms.
- Why is it important to **understand** the meaning of these concepts?
- Spend a short time in **self-reflection** on ways to prevent harmful assumptions when showing love and compassion to people. Other terms to explore may include: *discrimination, prejudice, caste systems, microaggressions, implicit bias,* and *explicit bias.*

Term	Definition
Subculture	
Minority	
Ethnocentrism	
Stigma	
Stereotyping	
Generalization	
Others?	

Answers can be found at the end of the lesson.

The entry posture diagram (below), used for many years by InterVarsity Christian Fellowship in their Global Missions training, shows the ways to approach cultural differences without causing distress, frustration, and fear. It illustrates that when encountering cultural differences, a person has a choice to make. If a person follows the upper track, there will be openness, acceptance, and trust between people. This means observing behaviors—are people standing far from each other or very close together, who is served food first, and where do people sit—on the ground, on chairs, is someone given a seat of honor for age or education.

It also means observing the way people greet each other—is there a handshake, a bow, or kissing of cheeks? Are certain gestures taboo, such as the "ok" sign, or the "victory" sign used in Western cultures that have sexual meanings in other cultures? Are there words that may have different meanings depending on the place you live? You can always encourage people to show you the way they do things and have them explain why it is important in their culture. This will lead to rapport and understanding, as well as deepening relationships.

On the other hand, if a person follows the lower track of fear, suspicion, feeling superior and inflexibility, building relationships will be difficult, sharing the gospel will be limited, and this may result in frustration, confusion, tension, and even embarrassment or aggression (Elmer 2002). Self-reflection on personal biases, and asking questions to understand, will mitigate negative outcomes.

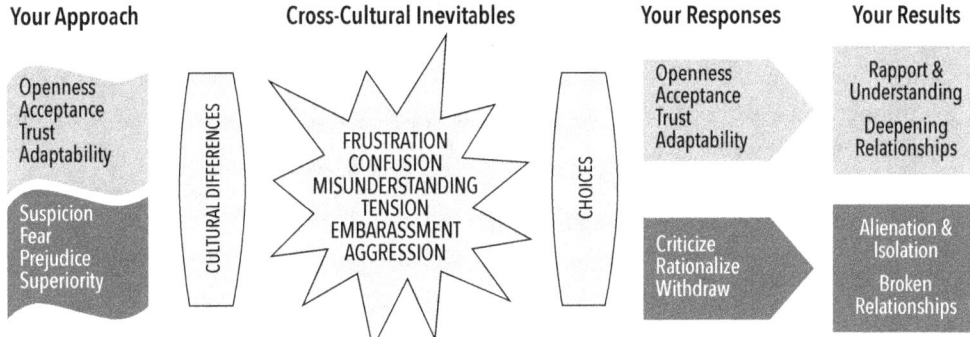

Figure 6: Entry Posture Diagram

This diagram is also referred to as the cultural adjustment map. Just because you may experience some of these feelings when working in a cross-cultural setting, it doesn't mean you are an immature disciple. It just means you are human and potentially need to put aside your implicit bias and rely on the Lord for his guidance.

For those going into a new culture or region for the first time, reflecting on this diagram may be very helpful as a reminder of ways to promote open communication. Think about your current, and future situation/location (either local or global) as you review the questions below:

Learning Activities

- **Reflect**—What is the difference between being open and being suspicious of different cultures?
- What kind of results will occur in a cross-cultural context if you **listen to others**? What if you are critical, superior, or fearful of other cultures?
- What are the best ways to **establish rapport and understanding** in a cross-cultural context?

Openness looks different in each country and region of the world. In many Western cultures, eye contact is acceptable while in other cultures, it may be rude to look someone in the eye, especially if they are an older person, or a different gender. Ways to be open include smiling genuinely, reaching out to people in appropriate ways, asking questions in a non-condescending way, engaging people, suspending judgment, being generous, and spending quality time with people.

Acceptance is part of the equation too. "Accept one another, then, just as Christ accepted you, in order to bring praise to God" (Rom 15:7). In this passage, the Roman

Christians were divided over cultural issues. Paul reminds them of the importance of love for one another to bring praise to the Lord. Jesus approached all people in love and grace while still holding them accountable to the truth, and he is our supreme example.

That means we all need to communicate with those the Lord puts into our path with honor, dignity, and respect. We all have inherent dignity and worth since we were all created in the image of God—*Imago Dei* (Gen 1:27). Strategies may include asking what will build trust (or a friendship) in this cultural context (which may be quite different than ours). For example, find out if people are invited over to share a meal in an informal way (many parts of the world) or more formal way (many Western cultures). Some cultures prefer "popping in" unannounced, and they would be welcomed with refreshments, and for others that would not be the preferred method of getting to know someone (Elmer 2002).

Fellow image-bearers of God deserve respect within their cultural framework, and it helps when trying to build bridges to his kingdom. Not respecting a person and their culture may result in shame, and Middle Eastern societies, for example, are sensitive to shame. When any member of the healthcare or ministry team functions within their own implicit bias, and provides spiritual, physical, or emotional care in a superior and prejudiced way, it can cause people to withdraw, resulting in cultural distress. This can lead to further alienation rather than understanding, especially in a cross-cultural context, and sharing the gospel becomes next to impossible.

Cultural Distress

Remember that culture may include ethnicity, socioeconomic status, ability or disability, age, education, and occupation or profession. Cultural distress is a newer concept in the literature and happens when cultural awareness and cultural humility are not practiced, resulting in an actual physiological stress response, and cortisol release, which may not even be recognized. It also results in a feeling of being "othered" and/or "marginalized" and/or made to feel inferior in some way (DeWild and Burton 2017). This is especially true when there is a perception of a power imbalance, or dominance, and one person, such as a healthcare worker or even a pastor, demonstrates a superior attitude toward people. These leaders within their context are almost always in a position of power, due in part to potentially having more education than those they are serving. Causing distress of any kind is not the way to demonstrate honor, dignity, and respect for fellow image-bearers of God.

Often, care recipients are in a vulnerable state, no matter where in the world they may be, and may be in pain, suffering spiritually or physically, spiritually oppressed, and/or emotionally distressed. The result is that the care recipient perceives the care has been delivered in a culturally insensitive way, which may lead to a perpetuation or perception of colonialism. This can severely impact people wanting to access modern, scientific medical approaches, and it may deter people from seeking evidence-based care in the first place. Many people seek local, culturally acceptable (traditional) approaches to health before seeking one based on science and modern medicine, and they can either receive good care or poor care. The goal for Christians is to provide whole person care, including spiritual care, which goes beyond traditional or modern medicine alone, and begins with building trusting relationships (Elmer 2006).

Culture Shock

If believers are planning on serving in a cross-cultural context or among the disadvantaged, even if that is within their own state, region, or country, there is the possibility of experiencing culture shock. Culture shock is a state of bewilderment or distress a person can experience when they are exposed to a new or unfamiliar physical, social, or cultural environment. It can affect people emotionally, physically, mentally, and/or spiritually. It usually occurs when two worldviews collide and values, thinking patterns, space and time, roles, customs, and different traditions create conflict within a person. Surface differences can become overwhelming and include smells, sights, sounds, and tastes.

There are stages of culture shock: a) honeymoon, b) uncertainty, c) adaptation, and d) acceptance. When you first enter a cross-cultural experience, there are feelings of excitement, however, that may soon be replaced with uncertainty and doubt. This is when it is so important to stay grounded in the Word, prayer, worship, and fellowship. As time passes, the things that may have bothered you will become more comfortable, especially if language learning is occurring. The process of acclimating to a new culture is gradual and may not be linear. Allow the Lord to work in and through your life as you adjust.

Adapting to a new culture may include some of the following activities—more information about language learning can be found in a later lesson (Elmer 2002):

- Learn key words and simple phrases.
- Wear local clothing (if appropriate, such a head covering for women).
- Smile (if appropriate).
- Do not make negative comments about the culture.
- Ask questions, observe, and listen.
- Eat local food (if it is safe).
- Spend time with locals just getting to know them.

Just like Christian healthcare providers care for people wholistically, preparing for healthy cross-cultural transition is important too for all members of the ministry team. Ways to mitigate some of the effects of culture shock include learning about the culture, planning for possible unforeseen circumstances, learning to be humble, and being flexible, since schedules and meetings often shift and change without notice. And the most important thing to do is prepare spiritually for the kingdom work to be done. Put on that full armor of God (Eph 6:10–18); it will be needed to keep the enemy at bay.

Learning Activities

- **Read**—DeWilde and Burton, "Cultural Distress: An Emerging Paradigm" (https://bit.ly/48MTR1j).

- **Review**—Entry Posture Diagram and questions (figure 6).
- **Reflect**—From the ideas presented, what are one or two implications that you draw from in putting cultural humility into practice?

Part 2—The Role of Worldview/Religion in Culture

It is important for the Christ follower caring for other people and sharing the gospel to understand the role of worldview and religion within each culture and ethnic group. The term "culture" is not the same as "worldview" rather, they are each influenced by the other. Worldview answers the questions of what reality is, what is a human being, where do we go when we die, how do we know what is right or wrong, what is the meaning of life, and where does disease come from (Pratt, Sills, and Walter 2014; Sire 2004). A person's or people groups' worldview guides choices that are made related to life, marriage, death, and religion.

Everyone has a worldview, with some people being more influenced by the supernatural, magic, and the unseen world, and others more by science and the material world. Lesson 9 will present more ideas about the seen and unseen world. Worldviews help people navigate through life, shape the way people see the world around them, and determine how they will live their lives (Hiebert 2008). According to Poplin (2014), "Worldviews are like operating systems on a computer except that they are in our minds...determining the range of thoughts we will entertain" (28).

> A 2-year-old believes he's the center of his world, a Secular Humanist believes that the material world is all that exists, and a Buddhist believes he can be liberated from suffering by self-purification. Someone with a biblical worldview believes his primary reason for existence is to love and serve God. (Tackett 2017, para. 4)

The content being presented in this lesson could be considered generic principles of culture and worldview; however, the reader is reminded that believers are to care for the whole person. Those who follow a biblical, or kingdom focused worldview believe in God as the creator of heaven and earth, who created humans in his image, and people are all part of God's plan and purpose. This gives believers hope during suffering in light of a redeemed future (Dockery and Thornbury 2002). As followers of Jesus, believers can bring that hope of the gospel, through health and healing and restoration of *shalom*, by sharing the Lord's plan and purpose for people among all tribes, tongues, and nations. "*Shalom* not only focuses on the vertical relationship between God and us, but also includes the horizontal relationship between human beings" (Tazelaar 2001, 7). Believers are tasked with sharing this good news with all nations, tribes, and tongues.

Some people may not realize the truth and reality of the one true God who is present in each culture around the world. He reveals himself through general revelation, which includes the beauty of his creation (Rom 1:20), humanity created in his image, although humanity has been distorted by the fall of mankind, and through history as the Lord has led kingdoms and people. He reveals himself through specific revelation through the Word (2 Pet 1:21; 2 Tim 3:16–17), and Jesus himself, who is the "exact representation and perfect imprint of the Father" (Heb 1:3). Jesus himself used cultural analogies in his parables, which is something the disciples and his followers would understand. Another example of a cultural analogy was when he took on the role of a servant and washed the feet of his disciples (Elmer 2006).

Well-known missionary Don Richardson used the phrase from Ecclesiastes 3:11, "...he has set eternity in their hearts..." to describe the idea of redemptive analogies, which are similar to cultural analogies. In one of his most well-known books, *The Peace Child*, he tells the story of two warring groups in New Guinea which had a mythology about a peace child; one child offered to another tribe, adopted by the tribe, and being used to stop war. Once the cross-cultural workers who were serving there understood the importance of this practice, the analogy became an important communication bridge which was used to communicate the gospel of Jesus Christ to this culture, starting a spiritual awakening within that tribal group.

Almost every culture has traditions, practices, stories, or other ways of thinking that include some basic kingdom truth, and if a person can find these within other cultures, these redemptive analogies can serve as a bridge to explain the gospel message in a culturally relevant way (Guzik 2020; Richardson 2005). For example, there is a tradition in Vietnam between warring groups that is like the *Peace Child* story, and most cultures around the world have a flood story.

When looking at how religion and worldview are interrelated, we need to look at three worldviews, the worldview into which we are born which influences our own thinking and behavior, the worldview of the culture with which we are interacting that may be different from our birth culture worldview, and the kingdom worldview as revealed in the Bible. The more people in a birth culture and people in a host culture adopt a kingdom worldview, the more they will appreciate each other's worldviews and come closer to God and a kingdom worldview.

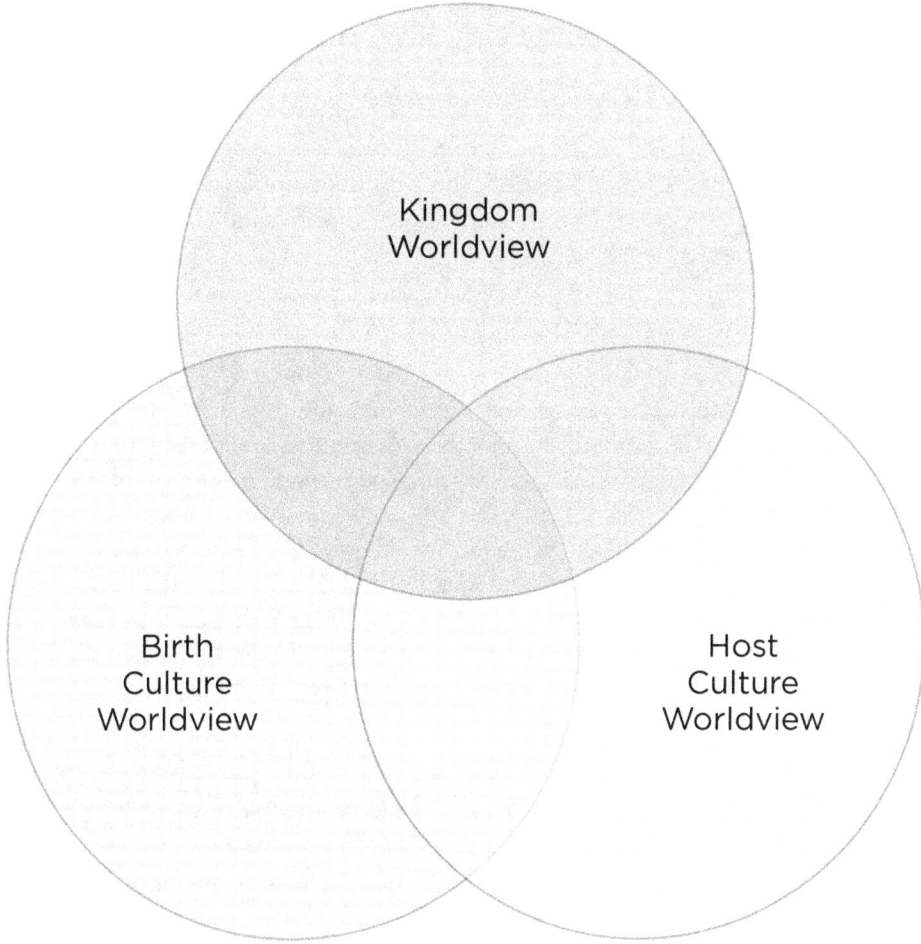

Figure 7: Worldviews

Part 3—Worldview Convergence

Birth Culture Worldview

When describing culture, worldview, and religions, it is important to examine different perspectives, and reflect on one's own view, since all people have a personal worldview, revere a particular religion, and hold certain beliefs. People think about themselves, and the world in a certain way. When a person grows up in a certain place, they learn the language, appreciate the food, music, art, and learn to live their daily lives in particular patterns.

It is important when working cross-culturally to examine one's own values and beliefs to become aware of one's worldview before interacting with people who have different cultures, worldviews, and religions (Pratt, Sills, and Walter 2014). This is helpful when trying to be culturally sensitive and have the right entry posture. It should also be noted that a person entering a new culture is often unaware that a practice is culturally determined until they have learned more about that culture, lived within that culture for a period of time, or learned the language.

The practice of giving a personal name is an example of a culturally determined practice. In some cultures, people are named by their parents, in others they are named by other family members, some cultures name their children by the day of the week when they were born, while other cultures may withhold naming a child until the child has reached a chronological milestone. The given names also follow culturally defined norms, such as paternal surnames, maternal ancestors, or clan names. A person coming from a culture where surnames are determined by the father's surname and thus identifies family relationships, one may find it difficult to determine family relationships in a host culture where this is not the practice.

Kingdom Worldview Revealed in Scripture

A kingdom worldview has been revealed in Scripture, is true, trustworthy, and guides believers. The metanarrative of Creation, the Fall, Redemption, and Restoration that has been presented in previous lessons is one way of viewing God's kingdom worldview. It begins with *shalom* and ends with *shalom*.

There are various presentations and discussions regarding the kingdom worldview that apply to healthcare and sharing the gospel. W. Meredith Long (2001, 118) wrote the following:

> Rev. Oscar Muriu, the pastor of our church in Nairobi, says that wherever he goes in Africa, he discovers a longing for the kingdom of God among its peoples. Essential characteristics of God's kingdom of *shalom* are shadowed in the holism of African traditional beliefs concerning health. Though covenants of health in the shadow "kingdoms" of African tradition are often shrouded with fear, the longing for healing and restoration is enlivened with every sickness or misfortune. Themes that emerge from traditional patterns of healing in Sub-Saharan Africa reflect the desire for healing that may only come fully through the powerful restoration of men and women in God's kingdom.

Throughout Scripture, it is very clear that the Lord's plan always has been to proclaim and demonstrate the whole gospel of the kingdom to the whole world (Rankin 2005). There are many tools and videos overseas workers have used to share the gospel message in a cross-cultural context, and the following video is one of them.

Learning Activities

- **Watch**—InterVarsity, "The Big Story Gospel Presentation" (https://bit.ly/3Swt0kA).

- **Reflect**—In what ways does this video uses the metanarrative of Creation, the Fall, Redemption, and Restoration to communicate the gospel message?

Host's Worldview/Religion/Beliefs

When working in a cross-cultural context, the host's worldview, religion, and/or beliefs may be completely different than a kingdom worldview. Instead of viewing other cultures and beliefs as wrong, see them as differences, which is a more neutral perspective. This will prevent believers from forming negative judgments and allow relationships to be built (Elmer 2002). There are many so-called labels given to different worldviews, religions, and beliefs, and it is helpful to have an idea of some of the practices and traditions associated with each one. However, to list all the many different worldviews and religions found around the world would be exhausting, so only a few will be discussed here.

Many people from different cultures will have a combination of beliefs and traditions, such as belief in spirits inhabiting rocks, trees, or rivers, which is common in animism and other faith traditions. In fact, animism is found in many forms around the world, sometimes in combination with other traditions. It is important when entering the host's culture to keep this in mind, that no culture has entirely one perspective. Even within a Western perspective, there are influences from other worldviews, such as the use of meditation and/or yoga (which came from practices in Hinduism and Buddhism). When going into another culture, it is important to remember that there is the possibility of both experiencing cultural differences as well as cultural similarities.

As early cultural anthropologists found, there are universal experiences people have such as birth and death (Hiebert 2008). Most cultures seek to answer basic human questions through their worldview and religion. Questions about meaning, purpose, life, death, and what people think is real, may be answered differently in a cross-cultural context. Another question may address whether there is one God, no god, or many deities. Hinduism for example, one of the oldest religions, includes a belief in up to 300 million deities and a vegetarian diet. If there is a belief in a "higher power," how is that deity (or deities) perceived? Or is this "higher power" a "supreme being" or something like a "conscience" or "force of nature"? Is this 'higher power' near or far away, controlling, or relaxed, and what form is this deity?

Other universal questions relate to the human status, as was mentioned earlier. What is a human being? What is the meaning and purpose of life? Are people just a bunch of highly diversified cells, and chemicals, which would be a scientific or naturalistic worldview, or are they a person created in the image of the one true God, which would be a biblical worldview? Other questions people may ask are: What happens to people when they die? Do they go to heaven, or are they reincarnated (Hinduism and Buddhism)? If a person believes a person is only cells and chemicals, they may not believe in heaven or any type of afterlife at all, and they will make life choices based on that perspective.

Other questions to consider are how do people know what is right or wrong? Does the host culture use the Bible, or another ancient text, or does the culture itself determine morality (Secular Humanism)? There are so many things that may be different in the host culture, and again, while it is impossible to know everything about every culture, it is helpful to learn about what the host culture does think or believe about these types of questions before serving within them (Sire 2004).

One of the important things for healthcare workers, pastors, and believers to consider when providing wholistic care, is asking a person what they think caused their disease, and where they think disease comes from. This helps better understand the perceived etiology of the disease. Mothers in Africa often explained their child's malnutrition as being caused by a curse put on the child by an ancestor, co-wife, witch doctor, or a jealous person.

Learning Activities

The following table is a grouping of some of the main worldviews/religions. Choose one or two worldviews that you are interested in and compare them to a biblical worldview. How are they different? How are they the same? A more complete fill in will be done in the next section. Refer to a book about worldview, or Sire, J. W. (2004), *The Universe Next Door: A Basic Worldview Catalog* (5th ed.), Downers Grove, IL: InterVarsity Press.

Worldview (based on Sire 2004)	Is there something greater than ourselves?	What is our place in the world?	Is there such a thing as absolute truth that provides guidance in decision making?
Christianity			
Naturalism			
Hinduism			
Buddhism			
Muslim			
Animism			

Using a non-formal education methodology such as the problem-posing method, can assist in learning about cultural understandings of illnesses. If a person thinks they are sick because of living a bad life, or because a shaman has put a curse or hex on them, they may follow a different course of action regarding their health than if they believe a pathogen or a nutritional deficiency caused their illness.

To promote spiritual, emotional, and physical health (*shalom*), it is important to think of culturally appropriate ways to motivate a people to possibly change their behavior. Knowing that people are often resistant to change, it is important to identify the ways they see themselves first (Fountain 1989). Second, it is important to identify potential barriers to caring for people with these different worldviews. Third, the obstacles need to be discussed with people while searching for ways to **bridge those gaps without alienating the person.** These bridges are often ways to share the gospel message (evangelism) and thus eventually to communicate and develop a kingdom worldview and lifestyle (discipleship).

Learning Activities

- **Read**—Matthew, Hockett, and Samek, "Learning Cultural Humility Through Stories and Global Service Learning" (https://bit.ly/3I6aTM1).
- **Reflect**—compare the listed worldviews with a biblical worldview. How are they different and how are they the same?

The chart below is another way of breaking down the worldviews of people. Healthcare providers are trained in the bio-medical, or scientific worldview. Some worldviews/cultures think it is important to keep everything in balance. The animistic worldview sees spirits in all objects and may have ancestor worship practices.

Bio-Medical, Scientific Worldview	Magical-Religious Worldview	Animistic Worldview	Kingdom Worldview
Often assume that all events in life have a material cause and effect, that the body functions like a machine, and all reality can be observed and measured. This view takes away the perspective that miracles can and do happen or that spiritual forces are at work.	The forces of nature must be kept in perfect balance (yin/yang, hot/cold Ayurveda) and breaking the laws of nature creates imbalances, chaos, and disease (Galanti 2015).	The world is an arena in which supernatural forces dominate and that the fate of the world depends on the actions of the supernatural world for good or evil. This perspective includes ideas about curses, ancestral intervention, or displeasure, and those holding this view may think that illness may be a sort of divine punishment	A kingdom worldview explains the origins of disease and suffering as coming from the fall. Because God is just, sovereign, and a healing redeemer, he at times allows ill health but is also all-powerful, able to redeem illness for his purposes and the person's benefit with a hope of eternal healing of all creation.

Glossary of Cultural Terms

Here are a few definitions of cultural terms. There may be other terms prevalent in your area—what are they and how are they significant?

Subculture refers to practices of groups of people who share characteristics that enable them to be identified as different from the main culture. They have their own set of ideas, interests, values, and behaviors while still operating within the bigger culture (McFarland and Wehbe-Almah 2015). Subcultures may be based on things like ethnicity, politics, occupation, sexuality, activity, and when one subculture has more power than another, they may be labeled as the "dominant" culture. (Galanti 2015)

Minority refers to a small group of people whose physical, ethnic, religious, or other cultural characteristics differ from the majority of people in a given society. The use of the term, however, may be discriminatory and people in the "minority" may be made to feel inferior, marginalized, and/or "othered." (McFarland and Wehbe-Almah 2015)

Ethnocentrism is a term from anthropology. It refers to an attitude and perception that one's own ethnicity or way of doing something is the best way. In this view, all other ways are inferior, unnatural, and may even be perceived as barbaric or "not as good." This can contribute to poor cross-cultural communication and causes cultural distress. The ideas in other cultures may be valid for them and inform their healthcare decisions and behavior. While we can never completely erase our ethnocentric ideas, being aware of our tendency can help us learn to appreciate other cultures. (Galanti 2015; Giger and Davidhizar 1999; Pratt, Sills, and Walters 2014)

Stigma is defined literally as a mark of disgrace, or a brand, made on the skin (Online Etymology Dictionary 2020). It is an attribute that is deeply discrediting. It is frequently met with prejudice, discrimination, stereotyping, and distancing, like the lepers in biblical narratives. This can result in barriers to people seeking care. Some people will not disclose health issues, such as HIV or domestic abuse, for fear of having a negative label placed on them.

Stereotyping is also a negative label, based on assumptions that all people are alike, and can lead to disrespect, discrimination, prejudice, and dehumanizing behavior towards individuals or groups (Bastable 2019; Giger and Davidhizar 1999). Stereotyping can be defined as an end point, where no effort is made to learn more, and may be perpetuated. In this situation, no attempt has been made to avoid future emotional, intellectual, or cultural understanding. Nor has any attempt been made to learn whether the person fits the preconceived statement, assumption, bias, or idea. Due to the amount of variability even within cultures, stereotypes are often wrong and may have unfavorable results. (Galanti 2015)

Generalization, on the other hand, is usually a more positive way to help a person understand other cultures in broad and general terms. It is defined as a starting point, which can help a person identify broad trends within cultures. However, in the course of time, more information will be needed about the culture to make an assessment to prevent oversimplification of values, behaviors, and patterns. (Dayer-Berenson 2011; Galanti 2015)

References

DeWilde, C., and Burton, C. (2017). "Cultural Distress: An Emerging Paradigm." *Journal of Transcultural Nursing* 28(4): 334–41.

Dockery, D. S., and Thornbury, G. A. (2002). *Shaping a Christian Worldview: The Foundations of Christian Higher Education*. Nashville: TN: Broadman and Holman Publishers.

Elmer, D. (2002). *Cross-Cultural Connections: Stepping Out and Fitting In around the World*. Downers Grove, IL: InterVarsity Press.

Elmer, D. (2006). *Cross-Cultural Servanthood: Serving the World in Christlike Humility*. Downers Grove, IL: InterVarsity Press.

Fadiman, A. (1997). *The Spirit Catches You and You Fall Down: A Hmong Child, Her American Doctors, and the Collision of Two Cultures*. New York: Farrer, Straus, and Giroux.

Fountain, D. (1989). *Health, the Bible, and the Church*. Billy Graham Center: Biblical Perspectives on Health and Healing.

Galanti, G. (2015). *Caring for Patients from Different Cultures* (5th ed.). Philadelphia, PA: University of Pennsylvania Press.

Giger, J. (2017). *Transcultural Nursing: Assessment and Intervention* (7th ed.). St. Louis, MO: Mosby-Elsevier.

Guzik, D. (2020). Text Commentary Related to '*Kingdom*'. Retrieved from blueletterbible.org.

Hiebert, P. (2008). *Transforming Worldviews: An Anthropological Understanding of How People Change*. Grand Rapids, MI: Baker Academic.

Long, M. (2001). *Health, Healing, and the Kingdom of God*. Wheaton, IL: Regnum Books International.

McFarland, M., and Wehbe-Almah, H. (2015). *Leininger's Transcultural Nursing: Concepts, Theories, Research, and Practice* (4th ed). New York, NY: McGraw-Hill.

Poplin, M. (2014). *Is Reality Secular? Testing the Assumptions of Four Global Worldviews*. Downers Grove, IL: InterVarsity Press.

Pratt, Z., Sills, D., and Walters, J. (2014). *Introduction to Global Missions*. Nashville, TN: B and H Publishing Group.

Rankin, J. (2005). *To the Ends of the Earth: Empowering Kingdom Growth, Churches Fulfilling the Great Commission*. International Mission Board.

Richardson, D. (2005). *Peace Child: An Unforgettable Story of Primitive Jungle Treachery in the 20th Century*. Ventura, CA: Regal Books.

Sire, J. (2004). *The Universe Next Door: A Basic Worldview Catalog* (4th ed.). Downers Grove, IL: InterVarsity Press.

Tackett, D. (2017). *What's a Christian Worldview?* Focus on the Family.

Yeager, K., and Bauer, S. (2013). *Cultural Humility, Essential Foundation for Clinical Researchers*. Applied Nursing Research 26(4): 1–12.

Reflection Questions for Group Discussion

This section has presented a starting place for reflection and conversation since there are often overlaps between different worldviews. Review the questions prior to the meeting.

1. What are the best ways to establish rapport and understanding in a cross-cultural context?

2. What techniques could be used to build bridges using redemptive analogies from the local worldview to a kingdom worldview?

3. Give examples of how worldview, beliefs, and values shape a person's behavior that can then impact their health.

4. What are the differences between these four categories of worldviews? Are there truths in each? Are there any similarities?

5. What is the dominant worldview where you are currently living?

Lesson 8
Cultural Factors Impacting Health

Summary	Knowledge Objectives
Culture influences everything, including a patient's definition and perspective of health. It also influences a patient's definition and perception of illness, whether they will self-treat their illness, or seek help from traditional healers. Culture influences how people behave when they are sick, who is expected to care for them (perhaps a shaman, diviner, herbalist, bonesetter, family, etc.), and where a person will spend their final hours (home or hospital).	1. Describe how culture impacts a person's understanding and behavior about health, disease, healing, suffering, dying, and death. 2. Evaluate the importance of a person's culture in healthcare decisions and behaviors. 3. Examine the concept of the "excluded middle" and how it impacts healthcare.
Thematic Content	**Attitude Objectives**
• The impact of culture on healthcare decisions and behaviors. • Ways of dealing with disease, suffering, and death within different cultures. • Coping with disease and healing in the perspective of God's kingdom. • Ways to gain insight into cultural beliefs and practices different than our own.	1. Demonstrate an understanding of cultural self-awareness regarding views and practices of health, healing, suffering, death, and dying in light of biblical teaching. 2. Express appreciation for Christ's example of breaking down cultural norms in his healing practice.
Conceptual Thread—Culturally Determined Factors	**Practice (Skills) Objectives**
These factors can include, but are not limited to an understanding of fatalism, language, customs, traditions, gender roles, dietary preferences, sexual practices, time orientation, routines, and expectations. Many cultural factors can be associated with occupation, education, income, and social status.	1. List healthcare practices in specific cultural contexts. 2. Tell how your personal story regarding health and healing are part of His story to build his kingdom (also called storytelling).

Part 1—Cultural Factors Impacting Health

Western medicine and healthcare often focus more on preventative and curative measures, while traditional/folk medicine is often more wholistic, focused more on the person than on the science. There are culturally determined factors that impact a person's understanding of health, illness, and life, such as relationships, fate, control, and time. How a person defines health and illness is shaped by many cultural factors and for some, may be viewed as a balance between the individual and the environment. The following sections will help explain some of these cultural factors for healthcare workers, pastors, and others who want to share the gospel and their lives among those in need across cultures.

Achieved Status and Ascribed Status

Western thinking values equality and opportunity for all people, no matter where or when they are born. However, in some cultures, people are born into a position in society and will never be able to change that place. This ties into the concept of fatalism, the next term presented in the lesson. There may be a 'pre-destined' group who are considered royalty or a caste or class system in other locations. Greetings in some places are different for those who are elderly, and respect is always shown whereas in other cultures, there are "untouchables"; people who are not considered worthy of respect or dignity or even being spoken to or touched by a person in a higher class. This is contrary to biblical thinking, where all people are made in the image of God, and all are worthy.

Take a place like Thailand for example, where the greeting of others is dependent on status; the placement of hands (high or low in the *wai* greeting) as well as the depth of the bow is determined by a person's position in life. Sometimes people casually hand out business cards, however, business cards can show status, and should not be treated casually or dismissed. Even the way the card is held and given to another person is important. Status and protocol are seen in places like China, where a middle status person would not be placed at the head of the table, but a professor or doctor would be asked to sit at the head of the table. People in other cultures may ask personal questions about a visitor's family and even financial situation to determine what the visitor's status is and how to treat that visitor. This may contribute to culture shock, that was discussed in the previous lesson.

Fatalism

Within some cultures, the idea of fate, which can be found in ancient Greek, Roman, and Norse mythology for example, is still prevalent. Fatalism guides the decisions people make, or do not make, about their health. People with this perspective may think that life "just happens," is determined by fate, and people are powerless to change anything now or in the future. This also means a person with this worldview may believe that all events are predetermined. People with this perspective may not ask for pain medication, thinking the discomfort is the will of God, or what will be, will be (*què serà serà*). Some may even embrace pain and suffering as a *karmic* debt and a means to earn a better "next" life.

The gospel addresses fatalism but underlying it all is God's intention to establish a righteous kingdom where one day there will be no more conflict, corruption, pain, and death. According to research done by Maercker, et. al. (2019):

> Fatalism can more generally be defined as the propensity of individuals or groups to believe that their destinies are ruled by an unseen power or are played out inevitably rather than by their will. The concept of fatalism has been closely intertwined to the development of religious and philosophical thought. Thus, it is not surprising that the precise meaning of the term fatalism changes across cultures and historical eras.
>
> Some authors have pointed out that different types or variances of the term can be distinguished: notably neutral and pessimistic… Neutral or non-judgmental fatalism is thus the belief of not being able to influence, regardless of whether something good, something bad or something indifferent happens. Pessimistic fatalism, on the other hand, is the expectation that nothing good will happen, but that all human impulses will fail sooner or later. (p. 2)

Internal or External Locus of Control

Another factor influencing the decisions people make about their health is their locus of control, which is a term first used in Social Learning Theory (Rotter 1966). Evaluating locus of control helps explain what people may think about their life experiences. Like fatalism, those who have an external locus of control believe there are external forces which are beyond their control influencing the outcome of events in their lives.

This means people may be more resigned to accept unfavorable health conditions and may not expend as much effort in health promotion or disease prevention strategies. They may believe compliance with medical treatment and health are unrelated, so they may be unmotivated to change their behaviors. On the other hand, a person with an internal locus of control feels they can control their environment, there is a relationship between compliance and health, and they are more likely to take actions to promote their health. Their focus may be more on self, rather than others, and they may experience actual physical discomfort when they feel there is a lack of control.

Time Orientation

Historically, industrial cultures focused on the importance of being on time to work, earning sick time, and not losing time (a focus on productivity). Time became an important factor in everyday life. A focus on the future also became important in this context as products were built and planned to meet future economic goals. The focus on time became even more stressful as technology and advances in science refined the concept of time to nanoseconds instead of minutes (Elmer 2002).

Because of this background, people raised in Western cultures and healthcare providers in that context often view time as extremely important, however, there are some places around the world where there is only a distinction between night and day, meals, and sleep. Responding to a family matter may be more important than meeting at a scheduled time for an appointment. Some cultures emphasize the past, some the present, and some the future. This difference can also have an impact on whether people seek healthcare in the first place.

For example, agricultural cultures may not be as worried about minutes, rather, they may focus on seasons. The idea of time is more fluid, as crops are planted, and the quality of unfolding events is the primary concern. There may also be a focus on building relationships and the occasional friend stopping by to talk. Biblical culture refers to *chronos*—segments of time, or a time period. In the Old Testament, time was sometimes viewed as prophetic as the Jewish people looked to the coming of the Messiah. The other word that is used is *kairos*, which can be translated as the right time, an opportunity, or meaningful time, demonstrating value of each moment, whenever it will occur (Elmer 2002).

Those with a past-time orientation are often very traditional, have done things the same way for generations, and often accept traditional or alternative approaches to medicine. People with a present-time orientation may be less likely to use preventative health measures, especially if they feel fine. On the other hand, people with future-time orientation may embrace preventive measures, new therapies, change, and progress. It is important to determine whether a person's time perception is due to cultural phenomena or a biochemical or psychological cause.

Part 2—Cultural Influences on Healthcare Decision Making Case Study

Ngoc Ly, a twenty-five-year-old Vietnamese man, was hit by a car while riding his bicycle to work. Paramedics were able to resuscitate him, but the physician at the local trauma center determined that Mr. Ly was clinically brain dead. He placed him on life support until the family could be notified.

When the family arrived, an interpreter explained Mr. Ly's condition to his wife and parents. They nodded in understanding and quietly left the hospital. Normally, the staff neurosurgeon would then have pronounced

Mr. Ly dead and removed him from the ventilator, but he was suddenly called to surgery.

Later that afternoon, Mr. Ly's family met with Dr. Isaacs, the physician they had spoken to earlier. Dr. Isaacs intended to tell them of the plan to pronounce Mr. Ly dead and discontinue the ventilator, but the Lys had other plans. They informed him that they had consulted a specialist who said this was not the right time for him to die. Dr. Isaacs was confused. What kind of specialist would make such a recommendation? As it turns out, an astrologer who had read Ngoc Ly's lunar chart advised the family that his death be postponed until a more auspicious date.

The physician had never encountered a situation like the one now facing him. Fearing legal repercussions if he did not abide by the family's request, he agreed to keep Mr. Ly on life support until further notice. A little less than a week later, the Lys called to tell him that Ngoc could now die. (Galanti 2015, 203–4)

Learning Activities

- **Reflective question**—What are your thoughts after reading this scenario?
- What culturally determined factors may have been at play?
  Be prepared to share as you are together as a group.

Individualism vs. Collectivism

When interacting with people of other cultures, it is important to consider the ways decisions are made within the culture; are decisions made by the individual, a leader of the household, a spiritual or religious leader, or the family members. One-way decisions, seen in mostly Western contexts, are approaches based on individualism. People who have this perspective are focused on personal identity, individual rights, and personal needs. There is an attention to self-efficacy, individual responsibility, and an "I" rather than "We" mentality.

People with this perspective may value individual goals and achievements over group goals and feel that each person is responsible for their own decisions and actions. There is also the perspective that speaking one's mind is a good attribute that reflects honesty and integrity. Some cultures may be task-oriented, assertive, and very outspoken. A person from another culture may not agree with a suggestion; however, they may go along with the idea—it is better to encourage people to show you their way instead (Elmer 2002; Hiebert 2008).

> *If you want to travel fast, go alone.*
>
> *If you want to travel far, go together.*
>
> —African proverb

This proverb is a good example of the different ways people might think about traveling on this life journey—together versus alone. The "together" mindset is called collectivism. This perspective values the relationships within a group, cohesiveness, and collaboration among people. Harmony is important to maintain, as well as building relationships—developing relationships is more important than the task, although the task will eventually get done. A person with this perspective will prioritize the group over self and a person's identity may be dependent on where they were born and what role they have within the group (Hiebert 2008). This becomes important when providing information to people, who may or may not want to know about their own health and illness, and/or make decisions about potential treatment options.

North Americans traditionally value doing their own thing and having it their own way in many decisions and life choices. Other cultures around the world are focused more on the larger group, and do not function independently. This way of thinking impacts both health behaviors and understanding and responding to the gospel—those who live in a collective culture may need to consult family members for permission to follow Christ. A strategy that may work in a collective context would be visiting a whole family, not just one member, to build trust and establish a relationship before sharing the gospel (Elmer 2002).

Linear vs. Circular Thinking

Linear thinking is very "Western" with a starting point, which comes very early in any conversation, and an ending point. People may become impatient when it takes a long time for the person speaking to come to the point. Curved thinking, or indirect communication, may start with a more peripheral idea, and then very slowly, layers are peeled back in the conversation to the main idea in the middle, or heart of things, provided trust has been established along the way. If trust has not been established, the heart of the situation or problem may not be uncovered.

In African countries, for example, pastors may talk in what is known as a flower petal pattern. They start with a point, verse, or focus, veer out from the main point, and come back, repeatedly, to the main verse or point. For Westerners, this may seem repetitive, but it can be very effective and allows people to remember what was emphasized in the discussion (Elmer 2002). Some Latino cultures use a deductive approach, and may rely more on things such as intuition, emotions, and feelings.

People may think about choices in their health in either a linear or circular way as well. People within some cultures make decisions about life, health, and death in a linear fashion, especially those within a Judeo-Christian worldview (Sire 2004). Decision making is taken one step at a time. Once one item is addressed, those with linear thinking move on to the next item.

However, in circular thinking cultures, people make health choices differently. All the items and options are presented before a decision is made. Often, decisions are implicitly understood in circular thinking, and may not be evident to a linear thinker. For those circular thinkers who also have reincarnation as part of their belief system, this perspective allows for people to be fatalistic in their choices, since the person may think if things don't work out, they may get another chance in a "new life." It is important to understand how people think and make decisions.

"Normal" vs. "Abnormal" Health

Each culture defines what is normal differently. It is considered normal for people to wear eyeglasses if they have difficulty visually focusing. It's not necessarily considered a disease. Many people have this problem, and it is easily corrected. In some cultures what we ourselves may consider pathology is considered normal. In other cultures, not being able to see well might be a "normal" part of everyday living, especially when getting old. Likewise, having a bit of diarrhea every now and again, may be considered normal, because it happens to so many people every day. Poor eyesight or diarrhea may not be considered something that needs to be dealt with medically in some regions of the world. In some places, having seizures is seen as "normal" and means that person is in touch with the supernatural. Pregnancy is another situation that one culture may view as normal, and not seek any medical treatment, even birthing children in the bush, whereas other cultures go in for regular visits throughout the pregnancy. Review the chart below—compare the different perspectives.

Learning Activities

- **Reflect**—What do people think causes their disease where you are serving?
- Why do people think there is suffering in the world based on their worldview?
- What are the implications for caring for non-Christians based on the chart below? Fill it out as much as possible, and it can be used in discussion.

Worldview (based on Sire 2004)	Does God exist in this worldview? Yes or no? If yes, one or many?	What is a human being? Cells and chemicals? Created being? Other?	What happens to a person at death? Is there a heaven? Reincarnation? What death rituals are practiced?	How do people know what is right and wrong (ethics)? Are there rules or guidelines?	What potential barriers to healthcare may occur with this worldview?
Christianity					
Judaism					
Islam					
Naturalism					
Nihilism					
Existentialism					
Hindu					
Buddhism					
Animism					

Part 3—Cultural Ways of Dealing with Disease, Suffering, and Death

Disease

Diseases arise from a variety of sources. Look back on the assignment called the *Many Causes of Disease* (from Lesson 2). Based on cultural views and practices, and despite many advances in science and medicine, people around the world still have different views on the cause of their illness. There is an element of truth in all the different beliefs—there is a relationship between health and behavior, the environment can be a factor, illness can be due to negative mental processes, diseases have natural causes, or result from spiritual oppression, and sometimes, a disease may have no discernable origin.

Those trained with a bio-medical focus have the perspective that many diseases have a biological cause. When using that lens, many emotional, social, spiritual, and cultural "causes" of disease may be ignored or not valued. For example, according to the practice of Ayurveda, a system of medicine practiced in India, is based on the idea that disease is caused by an imbalance or stress in a person's consciousness. All ailments in this perspective, mental or physical, are caused by the imbalance of the *doshas*, or energies. According to those who practice Ayurveda, endogenous causes of the disease include internal variations of the *doshas*, and exogenous causes refer to injuries caused by factors from outside. If someone follows this belief system, they may not adhere to Western medical practices. That is why it is so important to enter cross-cultural situations in an open way to discover the traditional practices that may be used related to health and disease.

Suffering

Suffering is a universally lived experience. Refer to the reading in Lesson 2 about suffering. According to Dr. Daniel Fountain (1989), every religion and culture has wrestled with the concepts of suffering, disease, and death. Not all suffering can be overcome, nor can all diseases be cured, although God does continue to allow for miraculous healing at times. The word suffering comes from *sofrir*, which means to bear, endure, resist, permit, tolerate, allow to occur, or fail to prevent (Etymology Dictionary 2019). But in the biblical view, suffering produces perseverance, character, and hope (Rom 5:3–4).

Suffering includes pain, misery, anguish, or distress that is caused by injury, illness, or loss, which can be felt physically, mentally, or emotionally. Suffering involves an experience or sensation that is perceived by a person as painful or harmful and causes overwhelming distress in their whole being. Suffering and pain are often described together, but research shows suffering can have psychological, spiritual, and social causes as well. Part of the suffering and growing process in life according to some researchers is that growing through suffering can be seen as a coping response, when a person begins looking for the cause of their problem or pain and doing something about it (Arman and Rehnsfeldt 2007).

True healing can only come when a person has been restored to wholeness, *shalom*, which includes his peace, tranquility, quiet, rest, security, justice, contentment and soundness of mind, body, and spirit in the context of relationships with God, self, other people, and creation (Shelly and Miller 2006). While it is important to address the physical causes of suffering and disease, it may also be a time for learning about who God is and growing in faith. It is important for Christians to be a light of Christ, show compassion, listen, and reflect him to those who may not know him no matter where they are serving. We can't always understand God's ways.

> The explanation of Job's suffering is the fact that God and Satan had made a battleground of his soul. It was not for Job's chastening or his perfecting, but for an ulterior purpose which he did not know, but his intuition made him stick to the fact that the only One who could explain the sublimities of Nature was the One who could explain what he was going through. (Chambers 1980, as cited in text commentary from blueletterbible.org)

In fact, pain can, at times, be considered a blessing as it alerts a person that there is something wrong and needs attention. Paul Brand, the famous missionary surgeon whose sentinel work in leprosy, and later in diabetic neuropathy, pointed to the usefulness of pain in preventing the progression of disease.

Through biblical revelation, God has shown humans that he is good, and he gained the victory over evil and death through the cross and resurrection. He has chosen to redeem every tribe, tongue, and nation from sin and to accomplish his global plan and purpose through his people. While suffering is difficult, believers can offer hope by caring for others who are suffering; in this way they work toward restoration of wholeness, or *shalom* (See Lesson 1 on *shalom*, suffering and salvation.) Prayer in the midst of suffering is key, which starts by acknowledging the Lord is sovereign. God has a purpose in the suffering of his people and the healing that they bring: "We know that in all things God works for good with those who love him, those whom he has called according to his purpose" (Rom 8:28).

Death

There is nothing hidden from God—everything, even the realm of the dead and depth of the sea is naked before him (Job 26). The rituals associated with death and dying vary across the globe, based mainly on worldview, and those without hope of heaven may have the added burden of no hope beyond the grave. When serving in a cross-cultural context, there may be limited resources for dying people, such as palliative care or hospice, so a focus on spiritual care and comfort for those who are lost is even more important. It also requires appropriate familiarity with those being cared for and their cultural perceptions. Shelley (2000) identified three spiritual needs that all people have in addition to the need for a personal relationship with God. They are 1) the need for meaning and purpose in life, 2) the need for forgiveness, and 3) the need for love and belonging.

Careful assessment of a person's worldview and the spiritual needs that are presented by the person are foundational for providing appropriate spiritual care. While Christians need to be ready to demonstrate and proclaim the good news to the dying, it is also very important to listen first to those who are suffering, and dying, and assess their readiness to receive that message. Believers need to be careful about whose needs we are meeting—ours to present the gospel or the person whom God has entrusted to our care.

When people have different worldviews about end-of-life care, it can make caring for them challenging. Often, people from different cultures may not want their loved one to know that they have a life-limiting diagnosis, so communication challenges may occur. In individualistic societies, it is thought that people should be allowed to make their own autonomous decisions, which may be a much different viewpoint than those from a group-oriented mindset (collectivism) may hold. Healthcare providers and pastors in this situation can preserve the sacredness of life, which includes cultural sensitivity in the process of death and dying.

When people are given a potentially life-limiting diagnosis, it is often a terrifying situation, especially if they do not believe there is anything beyond death. For those who do not believe in heaven and the resurrection, it may be a time of fear. This may provide the perfect opportunity for a believer to bring in a biblical perspective of who Jesus is, his perfect love, and his saving grace. Understanding the importance of death beliefs and rituals can help not only show the love of Jesus but also may serve as a bridge to the gospel. Rituals vary, for example, practicing Hindu's may prefer to die at home, the eldest son is responsible for ritual planning, and the body is usually cremated. Some cultures prefer burial within 24 hours, such as the Islamic and Jewish faith traditions.

All believers are called to serve and meet the needs of hurting, vulnerable, broken, and even dying people. As was mentioned in the previous lesson, believers need to be clothed with humility—putting on the apron of service just as Jesus did before washing the disciple's feet (1 Pet 5:5; John 13:4). His purpose was, and is, for all things to be reconciled to himself (2 Cor 5:19; Eph 2:16; Col 1:20, 22; Phil 2:10), to be loved, served, and worshipped by people from all nations. Christian believers can use their gifts, talents, and skills, to overcome evil, perhaps even perform miracles, and become a blessing to others.

> You are the light of the world. A city on a hill cannot be hidden. Nor do people light a lamp and put it under a basket, but on a stand, and it gives light to all in the house. In the same way, let your light shine before others, that they may see your good works and give glory to your Father who is in heaven. (Matt 5:14–16)

All this reminds us that the Lord has ultimate authority over sickness and health. The story of the centurion in Matthew 8:5–13, reminds us that even though the man's servant was dying, he believed that the Lord could heal him. Jesus was amazed at the faith of the centurion, and because of his faith, he was invited into the kingdom of God. We can learn to proclaim the gospel to all tribes, tongues, and nations from his word, through our witness, and as we pray (Fidler 2020).

Other Factors to Consider

When working and serving in a cross-cultural environment, either locally, or globally, it is important to understand many factors that have been presented in this lesson. For the goal driven person—the "mission" is defined in terms of tasks and checklists—language, translation, evangelism, church planting, discipleship, healthcare, and more. These folks are hardworking, however, sometimes there is less value on building relationships. The relational person—who focuses on nurturing relationships will find that socialization helps the goals get done, and the job may not get done if trust is not established as we saw in the last lesson in the Entry Posture Diagram. If the relationship is not built first, believers may be heard as a "clashing symbol" (1 Cor 13:1). According to Elmer (2002), task-oriented people often focus only on the Great Commission (Matt 28:19–20). The Great Commandment to Love needs to be the focus for believers as well (Matt 22:36–40).

Learning Activities

- **Read**—Tazelaar, G. (2009) "Embracing Shalom: Moving into Fullness of Life" (https://bit.ly/3vQN7B2).
- **Reflect**—what are the spiritual needs a person in the host culture might be experiencing?
- After reading Grace Tazelaar's article "Embracing Shalom," reflect on the "Entry Posture" diagram again to determine what spiritual needs a person in the host culture might be experiencing. Be ready to share your thoughts with the group.

Part 4—Practical Ways to Gain Insight into Cultural Beliefs and Worldviews

Jesus was very familiar with the cultures of the people he came to save. He made his teachings relevant to his audience and used examples in his stories they would understand. He talked about fishing with the fishermen and farming with the farmers; and he related to the Roman centurion in a different way than the Jewish religious leaders. Believers can communicate acceptance of people who have different views by honoring and respecting them. "God blesses people, people bless each other, and people bless God" (Elmer 2006, 62). The point of believers being blessed is to bless others. Those who are blessed to be a blessing, as Abraham was blessed to be a blessing in Genesis 12:1–3, need to able to build bridges in practical ways by understanding different worldviews so they can lead non-believers to an understanding of the kingdom worldview.

Storytelling

Stories are a basic component of the human experience used around the world to share beliefs and experiences. When approaching healthcare missions, especially in areas where there is low literacy, high orality, and storytelling is normative, it is helpful to use the oral story approach, "If you listen to me properly, I feel good" is often said by people who receive cross-culturally sensitive care. Listening to the factors that influence healthcare choices people make, will help guide patient care that is sensitive to cultural beliefs and practices. When providers (or pastors) don't listen to a person's story, even if it seems to be irrelevant in the moment, important details may be missed, and outcomes and relationships improve when people feel they are valued. Part of the ways cultural distress occurs is by not listening to and valuing a person's personal story.

When global health workers and pastors listen to a person's story and enter into it, accuracy in assessment can help tailor care and prayer to their cultural values and beliefs. This also shows the person respect, and honor, allowing the possibility for spiritual discussions to occur related to the Great Physician. As believers know, Jesus used storytelling in the form of parables to teach and communicate about God's kingdom. His teaching methodology—presenting a story, asking questions that helped the learner to own the knowledge and apply it to everyday living, is an example of nonformal learning and can be utilized in health education and community development.

In high technology areas, there has been a huge increase of the use of social media to tell a person's story. People are using social media to boost their businesses, reach others, and tell their story. This practice validates the importance of story, and storytelling with people from a variety of backgrounds. While the use of social media storytelling in a cross-cultural context is a relatively new frontier, there is the possibility that this method has the potential to enable health messaging and the gospel to be presented in culturally appropriate ways.

Learning Activities

- **Read**—Chaponniere (2010) "Facts through Fiction: Teaching Health by Telling Stories" (https://bit.ly/3vWjZIq).
- **Reflect**—What aspects of your personal story would you want to share with someone? Why do you think stories are so effective?

Narrative

To understand God's story, his mission for the church, and the church's mission to the nations, it is important to understand the biblical narrative. The Bible is a unified, grand narrative, including creation, the fall, redemption, and ultimate restoration as has been discussed in earlier lessons. It is written in a master narrative, or story format, something that many cultures around the world are comfortable with even if a postmodern world often discounts the idea of a meta-narrative. The gospel, or good news, is his story, his redemptive plan of salvation for lost and broken people living in sin. It is also a story of hope, as he brings us back into a right relationship with him.

Messengers of the gospel need to develop a deep understanding of the local culture, wherever they are working, and a genuine appreciation of it. Disciples are called to and commissioned to proclaim and teach the gospel to others, across cultures, to people of every language and tribe. The Lord is with his people as they go, he equips believers, and keeps his promises, as the stories of Joseph, Moses, Jeremiah and many others illustrate. Christians can integrate the gospel into conversations to creatively share his story with faith and courage, confident in his power.

An example of living out the Great Commission can be found in the life of Hudson Taylor, who amid great adversity, was able to completely surrender and depend on the Lord in all circumstances. Four of his eight children died in China as well as his first wife. Despite that, he still wanted to reach every province in China with the gospel, and his life in Christ was characterized by being humble, adapting to local customs, being devoted to the Lord, and knowing his perfect peace (Fidler 2020).

Language Learning

Another practical way to gain cultural insights is to learn the local language. Many cultures will be polite to those from other places. However, attempts at learning a new language are usually appreciated and often open doors that using a translator does not. Language learning can provide insights into the culture that come with understanding the etymology of words (the origin and meaning), the cultural contexts of literature and oral history, and humor. Learning the language allows better understanding, more empathy, and stronger spiritual connections.

It is important to try to learn the language and build that bridge so that the unreached can hear and accurately understand in their heart language the message of the gospel. Learning a new language is a life-long journey and according to Fidler (2020), it allows believers to joyfully share the gospel with their neighbors. He writes:

> As Great Commission servants of Jesus, we have the obligation, this fundamental desire to share his Word, an "intense fire in [our] hearts, trapped in [our] bones" (Jer 20:9) to proclaim the gospel to the lost around us in their language, so that they can understand it. I want to help fan this desire into a roaring flame through some encouraging, purposeful, and effective language learning perspectives and practices, which will help us go the distance in our Great Commission calling. (9)

Culture Impacts Health and Health Impacts Culture

Some cultural practices can be health promoting while other practices may be detrimental to health. Those that are not harmful and those that are helpful can be allowed to continue and encouraged. Other practices such as female genital mutilation, binding of women's feet in China, extraction of cuspid teeth in children experiencing diarrhea, are practices that diminish and threaten lives and need to be carefully challenged and changed through advocacy efforts. Deeply held beliefs and cultural practices require a great deal of cultural sensitivity and long periods of time before change can be expected to be fully accepted and implemented.

There are ways in which disease can also change culture. The HIV/AIDS pandemic in Africa changed many cultural practices. For example, lengthy funeral and burial practices had to change in villages that were losing large numbers of young adults. There were villages where everyone between the ages of 18 and 35 had died. The elders determined that not everyone in a village had to attend every village funeral because the children needed to have the healthy members of the village dig gardens and grow food or else there would be additional health problems related to hunger and starvation.

Cultural Considerations in Healthcare Ethics

It is helpful to identify underlying values when approaching ethical decision making. Culture can and does influence those values. Perhaps one of the fundamental Christian values is that humans bear the image of God, *Imago Dei*, and are therefore worthy of dignity and respect. This means that all human beings deserve to receive care regardless of their age, ethnicity, language, gender, socioeconomic status, or religious practices. Some cultures may place different values on humans based on these categories and consequently make different ethical decisions.

The value of human dignity also underpins the way healthcare approaches research and obtains informed consent. If human life is not valued or valued differently, then the door can be opened to unscrupulous experimentation without consent. For example, the human experimentation on Jewish people that took place in Nazi Germany in the twentieth century and the Tuskegee experiments were completely unethical. It may seem that this could not take place under today's practice standards; but it is easy to place the efficacy and urgency of research and/or treatment, especially in times of health crises, over the value of the human person, especially the most vulnerable, created in God's image.

Another value presented in the Bible is free will. Christians believe that God created humans with the ability to choose while God remains sovereign. They earnestly desire that all people choose to have a relationship with the Lord. Sometimes they overstep the God-ordained free will of the people they serve in their zeal to present the gospel message and promote health. People who are injured, sick, and possibly approaching death are in a vulnerable and in an unequal power position with healthcare professionals and pastors. The focus of a Christian's care must be on the person or population that God has entrusted to them. The call to proclaim the gospel must not interfere with the plan that God has for that person, nor should coercion to a Christian faith be used as a requirement to receive care. Christian healthcare providers and those living out and sharing the gospel to the ends of the earth can and should be open to hearing from God regarding the spiritual status of those in our care and be willing instruments of the Holy Spirit in sharing the truth of the gospel in all its fullness.

References

Chaponniere, P. A. (1985). "Facts through Fiction: Teaching Health by Telling Stories." *Journal of Christian Nursing* 2 (1): 27–29.

Comfort, R. (2008). *World Religions in a Nutshell*. Newberry, FL: Bridge-Logos Publishers.

Elmer, D. (2002). *Cross-cultural Connections: Stepping Out and Fitting in Around the World*. Downers Grove, IL: InterVarsity Press.

Elmer, D. (2006). *Cross-cultural Servanthood: Serving the World in Christ-like Humility*. Downers Grove, IL: InterVarsity Press.

Everts, D. (2012). *Go and Do: Becoming a Missional Christian*. Downers Grove, IL: InterVarsity Press.

Fidler, P. (2020). *1000 Cups of Tea: Gospel Fluency across Cultures*. Preston Fidler.

Galanti, G. (2015). *Caring for Patients from Different Cultures* (5th ed). Philadelphia, PA: University of Pennsylvania Press.

Hiebert, P. (2008). *Transforming Worldviews: An Anthropological Understanding of How People Change*. Grand Rapids, MI: Baker Academic.

Maercker, A., Ben-Ezra, M., Esparza, O., and Augsburger, M. (2019). "Traditional Cultural Belief Potentially Relevant to Trauma Sequelae: Measurement Equivalence, Extent and Associations in Six Countries." *European Journal of Psychotraumatology* 10. https://doi.org/10.1080/20008198.2019.1657371.

Myers, B. (1999). *Walking with the Poor: Principles and Practices of Transformational Development*. Maryknoll, NY: Orbis Books.

Poplin, M. (2014). *Is Reality Secular: Testing the Assumptions of Four Global Worldviews*. Downers Grove, IL: InterVarsity Press.

Pratt, Z., Sills, D., and Walters, J. (2014). *Introduction to Global Missions*. Nashville, TN: B and H Publishing Group.

Ridenour, F. (2001). *So, What's the Difference*. Ventura, CA: Regal Books.

Sire, J. (2004). *The Universe Next Aoor: A Basic Worldview Catalog* (4th ed). Downers Grove, IL: InterVarsity Press.

Storti, C. (2001). *The Art of Crossing Cultures* (2nd ed). Boston, MA: Nicholas Brealey Publishing.

Tackett, D. (2017). *What's a Christian Worldview?* Focus on the Family.

Tazelaar, G. (2001). "Embracing *Shalom*." *Journal of Christian Nursing* 18(2): 4–8.

Reflection Questions for Group Discussion

1. After completing the assigned reading and other assignments for this lesson, select at least four healthcare practices in specific cultural contexts you have learned about that you did not know before.
    a. Did anything surprise you? If so, what?

    b. What does this cultural group think about health and healing?

2. What aspects of your own personal faith story (or journey) related to any of the content covered in the curriculum so far would you want to share with someone so they could understand who you are and the ways the Lord has worked in your life?

3. Why do you think stories are so effective in communicating health information?

4. Write or give an example of a story or parable from Scripture that communicates an important aspect of wholistic healthcare.

Lesson 9
Culture and the Unseen World

Summary	Knowledge Objectives
It is important to understand the physical and the spiritual realms of the world—both what is seen and what is unseen. For many people, the unseen world is a place of fear and uncertainty. However, for the believer, the unseen world can be a place of hope, miracles, and his perfect peace (*shalom*).	1. Examine the overlapping concepts of the seen world, the unseen world, and the "excluded middle" and how they impact choices people make about their life. 2. Explore spiritual warfare, good, and evil in a cultural context. 3. Define culture-bound syndromes.
Thematic Content	**Attitude Objectives**
• There are guilt-innocence, shame-honor, and fear-power cultures around the world. • Shamans, witch doctors, and others engage in practices that are part of the unseen world. • Angels and demons are part of the world view of many world religions, including Christianity. • Spiritual warfare is real, and believers have the tools they need for the battle. • The Excluded Middle is where the seen and unseen world merge.	1. Evaluate cultural practices that may surprise the learner. 2. Examine the ways the enemy works within the world to deceive people.
Conceptual Thread—Powers and Principalities	**Practice (Skills) Objectives**
This phrase occurs six times in the KJV, and other versions of the Bible translate the words as "rulers and authorities," "forces and authorities," and "rulers and powers." The phrase refers to the evil spirits, or demons, that are in a spiritual battle in the unseen world against the people of God and the goodness of creation. These are described as strongholds, against which the kingdom of God will prevail.	1. Discuss guilt, shame, and fear as they relate to the biblical concept of sin in cultures around the world. 2. List ways one can confront the powers and principalities which may manifest themselves. 3. Pray for courage to engage in fighting disease and evil forces for the liberation of people and populations.

Part 1—Cultures Living in the Balance

When the fall occurred, and Adam and Eve chose to disobey the Lord, three things occurred—sin entered the world, resulting in guilt, shame, and fear. Many who serve in cross-cultural contexts find these three concepts helpful to understand as they navigate cultural differences. Many missiologists and cultural anthropologists would say that all cultures have these three elements embedded in their practices; however, some cultures may emphasize one of the three concepts more than the other. According to Pratt, Sills, and Walter:

> The cultures of the world tend to live on a balance of guilt-innocence, shame-honor, or fear-power. Western cultures that are more dichotomist in their orientation see people as either guilty or innocent. Asian cultures and most cultures embracing Islam have a high value of honor and avoid shame at all costs. Animistic cultures are constantly aware of evil spirits, ancestors' influences, magic, curses, and sorcery and live in fear of these or anyone who has the skill to manipulate their power. (2014, 141)

Guilt-Innocence, Shame-Honor, and Fear-Power Cultures

The division of the world into guilt-innocence cultures, shame-honor cultures, and fear-power cultures is generally traced back to the writing of Eugene Nida, and his anthropological textbook *Customs and Cultures* (1954). In it he writes:

> We have to reckon with three different types of reactions to transgressions of religiously sanctioned codes: fear, shame and guilt. It seems that for the most part people are afraid of being punished or of being caught in the act by some person or deity. Often there is a sense of shame, expressed as "I'd feel terrible if anyone saw me doing this." A sense of guilt expresses itself as an inner feeling of failure for not having lived up to what the society or deity expects, irrespective of whether one is caught or seen. This sentiment of guilt is far less common than might be supposed. Except for those neurotic persons who magnify their self-importance by self-incrimination, regarding oneself as guilty is not in keeping with man's egocentric way of life. Fear and shame are much more convenient attitudes for self-centered people. (150)

Within guilt-innocence cultures there is an internal sense of wrong, which influences beliefs and choices people make. Generally, Western cultures are more guilt-innocence based, and people know that they may be punished for bad behavior. There is more of a focus on the conscience of a person, and it is individualistic in nature. According to Lucenay (2019):

> Most guilt/innocence cultures are individualist (i.e., Western). We measure everything with the yardstick of right and wrong. We make laws that determine innocence and guilt. Knowing and exercising individual rights is a primary concern. We teach children to be law-abiding and expect them to develop a conscience. We define innocence as being right or as righteousness. People feel guilty for what they have done or not done. Communication is direct; confrontation is acceptable. (para. 6)

Shame-honor cultures exert external pressure within the culture by people or circumstances to conform. In shame-honor cultures, a person does not want to bring shame on themselves, their family, or even their country, and failure is the inability to meet their standards. It is preferable to bring honor to family and country. Lucenay states:

> Honor/shame cultures are generally collectivist. The issue isn't right or wrong but honorable or dishonorable. Acquiring honor and avoiding shame are the highest goals. Self-expression and fulfillment are less important than group success and honor. Shame comes from failing to fulfill the group's expectations. Individuals sacrifice for the good of the team, family, village, or country. Communication is indirect, and body language communicates feelings. The unspoken is as significant, if not more significant, than the spoken. (2019, para. 7)

Fear-power cultures are usually found in animistic contexts, where people are afraid of evil spirits, worship their ancestors, and will try to appease spirits through food, money, and other types of offerings. Lucenay writes:

> Fear/power cultures are also usually collectivist. People fear unseen forces such as evil spirits, curses, and ancestors. The goal is to appease or manipulate the spirits to act in your favor. The lion statues I saw [in Hong Kong] were symbols of power to scare away evil forces. (2019, para. 8)

In some Western circles, the guilt/innocence of mankind may often be emphasized more than the concept of shame/honor. The Apostle Paul uses guilt in Rom 3:19 (all the world is guilty before God—as lawbreakers) and shame in Rom 9:33 (believers will not be put to shame). Heb 2:11 and Heb 11:16 also focus on shame. Cozens (2018) has a slightly different perspective about the concepts of shame, fear, and guilt:

> … there needs to be greater *theological* investigation into the nature of shame and guilt. It is my contention … that shame is the default *primary* orientation, as experienced by Adam in Genesis 3, while—theologically speaking—guilt is produced by the experience of transgressing against a divine code, as Paul describes the Law in Romans 7. From this theological standpoint, it is shame which is the universal human experience; to then categorize the world—particularly the unevangelized world—into shame, fear and guilt cultures represents an unnecessary complication. (10)

No matter what perspective the reader may have, many people working in cross-cultural contexts agree that these concepts (guilt, shame, and fear) are a helpful starting point as they try to understand and serve where there are cultural differences. Understanding these concepts may help explain why people have certain practices they engage in, and an understanding of them may help the believer find a redemptive analogy (a practice or belief native to any given culture that distinctly parallels or illustrates the gospel, discussed in Lesson 7) to build bridges to the gospel (Richardson 2005).

Part 2—Intersection of the Seen and the Unseen World and the Place of the Excluded Middle

The Seen World

Science and discovery are amazing areas that the Lord encouraged mankind to explore when he commanded people to rule over and subdue the earth in the Great Cultural Mandate (Gen 1:28). During the Enlightenment, science became accepted as the main basis for knowledge and truth, and not the Word of God. People in many Western cultures have focused on the physical realm: what can be observed, quantified, and measured through the five senses and ignored or dismissed what is not observable, including much of the spiritual world. In fact, especially in healthcare, there is often an assumption that the spiritual and the physical aspects of care are separate concerns and only the physical aspects need to be addressed. This mindset has begun to permeate other cultures around the world who have embraced secular teaching, and it has even influenced the church. Sometimes, people are "spiritual" at church and then resume a focus on science, technology, and physical matters alone the rest of the week (Myers 2011).

In recent years some have tried to prove the existence of a spiritual world and its impact on health using scientific means such as studies to prove the efficacy of prayer or faith as a health intervention and a means to justify its practice. A quick search of studies and published work related to prayer and medicine conducted by the author of this lesson resulted in over 500 published articles in the CINAHL database and thousands of articles on a Google search. The underlying assumption even in these studies is that only that which is seen, and observable should be believed. Focus only on the seen world is not where the majority world lives, works, and plays, so the unseen world needs to be explored to better understand cross-cultural experiences.

The Unseen (Spiritual) World—A Place for Miracles

There is an interrelatedness between the seen and the unseen world, not always acknowledged, and this is where traditional medicine and other methods like spirit strings, curses, talismans, charms, and chants may be used to try to control the fear experienced by some people around the world (Myers 2011). Shamans and folk healers practice their rituals, and Ayurveda and Chinese Medicine are being used to treat people. The World Health Organization (WHO) defines traditional medicine as:

> The sum total of the knowledge, skills, and practices based on the theories, beliefs, and experiences indigenous to different cultures, whether explicable or not, used in the maintenance of health as well as in the prevention, diagnosis, improvement or treatment of physical and mental illness. (WHO 2022, para. 1)

As was mentioned, most people living in traditional cultures view the unseen world as very real and they may live in fear of what they cannot see (fear/power cultures). Likewise, many Christians do not separate the seen and unseen worlds. They believe that God is the Creator of both the seen and unseen worlds and is Sovereign over all. Christ-followers understand sacred revelation through Scripture, and it is a personal experience for each person. As Myers writes, "Loving God is spiritual work, and loving neighbors takes place in the material world" (Myers 2011, 7). Christians embrace the intervention of angels, value prayer, believe in miracles, and practice a variety of rituals such as anointing the sick or the exorcism of demons.

Addressing both the spiritual side and the physical or material side of caring for people wholistically is important when considering both individual and collective restoration and *shalom*. Trusting that Jesus has ultimate authority over everything, whether it is sickness, evil, sin, suffering, or death is important as believers depend on his strength, power, and peace. Cross-cultural work can be humbling as well as rewarding, however, the most important thing to remember is running the race well, with endurance, and being sustained by his strength alone (Fidler 2020).

The Place of the Excluded Middle in Global Health and Healthcare

Paul Hiebert called the place where the seen world and the unseen world intersect the **excluded middle** because it was not part of a modern naturalistic, bio-medical, or scientific worldview. Western thought focuses on science, cause, and effect, not on "superstition." If Christ-followers fail to take the excluded middle into account, they will not be able to understand the global community's perspective about the unseen world, resulting in not knowing how to answer questions about the other culture's thinking about that sacred space.

A biblical perspective is wholistic, where the physical and spiritual world is connected. "The fact that the Word became flesh explodes the claim that the spiritual and physical can be separated meaningfully" (Myers 2011, 8). In fact, in healthcare missions it is often a place where a host culture's worldview and the birth culture's worldview can find a common point of entry into a kingdom worldview, and perhaps also find that redemptive analogy to build bridges to the gospel.

Bryant Myers expands on this idea when he identifies the God of the unseen world as the gospel as Word (see the chart below). "In the beginning was the Word, and the Word was with God, and the Word was God" (John 1:1 NIV). Many cultures believe in other deities, and not the One True God. Myers presents the Excluded Middle as the gospel as Sign where miracles, angels, and signs and wonders take place. For the non-believer, the excluded middle is a scary place, and people live in fear, thinking that the spirits, shamans, and ancestors have power over their lives. For the believer, the excluded middle is a sacred, safe, and holy place. And finally, Myers presents the seen world as the gospel as Deed—where believers see the ways the Holy Spirit works in and through his people, not just the science and technology of our current times.

Modern Worldview		Kingdom Worldview	
Spiritual World 1. God 2. Allah 3. The Force 4. Christian Witness	Whose God is true? Gospel as Word	1. God the Father 2. The risen Christ 3. The saints before us	Unseen World
The Excluded Middle The domain of shamans and magic in traditional cultures	Whose God is more powerful? Gospel as Sign	1. Angels 2. Prayer and visions 3. Sacred space 4. Signs and Wonders	Unseen World
Seen World 1. Hear, see, feel, and touch. 2. Science and Technology	What Works Gospel as Deed	1. Holy Spirit with us 2. Christ in us 3. The Word of God 4. Science with a purpose	Seen World

Bryant Myers in *Walking with the Poor* 2011, 9. Adapted from Paul Hiebert, 1982.

Learning Activities

- **Review** the chart above.
- **Reflect**—Describe one thing you learned that you did not know before reading this section.
- Based on the chart above, what are the spiritual and healthcare implications when interacting with people from another culture, perhaps where you are currently working?
- **Describe** how you would connect the Christian worldview to another worldview in the area of the Excluded Middle in a healthcare context to create bridges.

Case Study

> **A Cambodian infant boy** was brought into the hospital diagnosed with dehydration 5 percent. His family practices Buddhism and have limited English. Mona, the nurse, examined the child's extremities, looking for a vein in which to start an intravenous line. She found one on the baby's arm. At that point, she noticed several strands of dark brown strings, about one-half inch wide, on both wrists. Mona prepared to cut the strings with scissors.
>
> Mrs. Tep, the baby's mother, walked in at that moment, looked horrified at what Mona was about to do, and began speaking loudly in her native tongue. Mona assumed she was upset because the infant was crying. But Mrs. Tep kept pointing to the strings; it was obvious that she did not want them cut. Mona did not understand what the problem was but communicated through gestures that she would not cut the strings. She then started an intravenous line in the infant's scalp. When the baby's parents saw this, the mother began to cry. (Galanti 2015, 88)

Learning Activities

- **Reflect**—Before moving on, stop and think:
    ◊ Why was the mother upset in the first place?
    ◊ Why was she upset about the IV in the scalp?
    ◊ What would you have done differently?
    ◊ What are the cultural/worldview implications?
- **Write**—a few ideas to share with the group.

The church has a role in the multicultural world with its fluid borders and everchanging situations. Believers can value all people and cultures since the Lord has placed and is at work in each family, tribe, nation, and tongue in their circumstances and locations. "The ministry of blessing can never be an ethnocentric affair; it must be a family affair, as in all the families of the earth" (Elmer 2006, 62).

Cultural Practices and Mystical Causality

After reading the scenario above, the reader may still have some questions. Some cultures think that if a hole is made in a baby's head, the baby's spirit or soul will leave the child and the child will die. Many cultures around the world tie strings around wrists or around other parts of the body. There are specific reasons for this depending on the culture, and it usually involves a ritual practiced by a shaman or witch doctor when the string is first tied onto the person. For some cultures, it is thought to be a way to shield the person from evil spirits and sickness, and those cultures live in fear of making the spirits angry. Other cultures think it helps keep the soul within the person and that they will stay healthy. It can also be used to bless someone at weddings, monk ordinations, graduations, and more.

Another interesting practice to explore is what happens to a placenta after a child is born. Some cultures think of the placenta as a twin of the child that has been born and it is worthy of full burial rituals. One idea is that the placenta is a spirit guide, another is that the placenta can connect the child to the land so they will never leave the place they are born, or another view is that the burial will help protect the child from harm in the future. Some cultures will wrap the placenta in a special cloth or leaves and bury the placenta in a particular place where it will be protected. Some of the cultural groups/countries that bury their placenta include, but are not limited to: Bali, Hmong Culture, Native Icelanders, Navajo People, Igbo Tribe of Africa, Maori of New Zealand, Japanese, and Chinese (Hollister 2018).

Another phenomenon that cross-cultural workers may want to understand is mystical causality. In some African and Asian cultures, sickness is thought to have religious, supernatural, spiritual, and mystical causes. This was presented in Lesson 7 as Magical-Religious thinking. For those who think this way, the world, relationships, pain, sickness, suffering, poverty, or wealth, and even death is all part of the mystery of life and cannot be explained in physical or even tangible ways. A person with this background may not think in what some might call "rational" or medically based ways, but rather, this person would want to consult the supernatural or spirit world using a spiritual healer. There are so many cultural practices that may be unfamiliar to the reader, and in this lesson, there is not enough time to cover them all. The authors again encourage learners to find out more about practices of specific cultural groups where they may be living and serving.

Part 3—Spiritual Warfare, Powers, and Principalities

The Adversary

Satan was a leader in the angelic world and led the revolt before falling away from God, taking his followers with him. The name "Satan" points to him as the "Adversary" of God. He enticed Adam and Eve, the crown of God's handiwork, and he seeks to destroy, and is therefore called Apollyon (the destroyer). After sin entered the world, he became Diabolos (the Accuser), accusing the people of God continually (Rev 12:10). He is represented in Scripture as the originator of sin (Gen 3:1, 4; John 8:44; 2 Cor 11:3). He remains the leader of the angelic hosts which he carried away with him in his fall and uses them to resist Jesus and his kingdom, and even to corrupt the natural world. He is called "the prince (*archon*) of this world" (John 12:31; 14:30; 16:11).

This does not mean that the adversary is in complete control, God is in ultimate control, and he has given all authority to Jesus, who came to destroy the work of the devil (1 John 3:8). Yet Satan is in control over the evil things that happen in this world and opposes the works of God's people. This is clearly indicated in Ephesians 2:2, where he is called "the prince of the powers of the air, of the spirit that works in the sons of disobedience." He is not human, but not divine, he has power, but is not omnipotent, he has influence on a restricted scale (Matt 12:29; Rev 20:2), and ultimately, he will be destroyed.

Jesus told his followers that opposition would occur in this world. The main source of that opposition is Satan, and the many evil demons who work against the kingdom of God in the unseen world that was just presented. This opposition is evident in many ways, some of which has already been discussed, and the difficulties that believers face are all part of a fierce spiritual battle. One of the strategies the enemy uses is to keep believers unaware of the fierce spiritual battle that is going on all around them. Sometimes, especially in a Western context, believers are led to believe that the spiritual battle is not important or can be attributed to something else. When serving in a cross-cultural context, that spiritual realm can become very apparent as non-believers battle against spirits, and consult shamans, which often allows them to be much more open to spiritual discussions and seek liberation from cycles of fear and oppression.

> For our struggle is not against flesh and blood, but against the rulers, against the authorities, against the powers of this dark world and against the spiritual forces of evil in the heavenly realms. (Eph 6:12)

Spiritual Warfare

The armor and weapons Christians have to fight against the spiritual strongholds, and the unseen powers and principalities are from God. They have divine power to demolish any strongholds the enemy might hold. Paul reminds believers that they are free from condemnation, and no matter what the circumstances are, nothing will separate a believer from the love of the Lord. That includes the evil that is present in the world. The key in sharing the gospel is to find a way to show his love within a spiritual battleground to those worshipping spirits, idols, or people instead of the one true God. Along with angels who are spirits sent to assist them, Christians have the Lord as the ultimate stronghold, refuge, and tower to face the battle.

> Who shall separate us from the love of Christ? Shall trouble or hardship or persecution or famine or nakedness or danger or sword? As it is written: "For your sake we face death all day long; we are considered as sheep to be slaughtered. No, in all these things we are more than conquerors through him who loved us. For I am convinced that neither death nor life, neither angels

nor demons, neither the present nor the future, nor any powers, neither height nor depth, or anything else in all creation will be able to separate us from the love of God that is in Christ Jesus our Lord. (Rom 8:35–39)

Good vs Evil

The enemy is perpetually at war with the followers of Jesus, and he has a multitude of demons working with him. Paul refers to this army as powers and principalities, who rule the darkness of this world—they are spiritual hosts of wickedness in high places (see Eph 6:12 above). Paul tells the believer that all our warfare is against "*spiritual hosts of wickedness.*" That is why he goes on to tell believers in the rest of Ephesians 6 to stand firm, stand in the strength of the Lord, and put on the full armor of God.

> Put on the full armor of God, so that you can take your stand against the devil's schemes. For our struggle is not against flesh and blood, but against the rulers, against the authorities, against the powers of this dark world, and against the spiritual forces of evil in the heavenly realms. (Eph 6:11–12)

The New Testament also shows the Lord being tempted when the enemy showed him all the kingdoms of their world in John 14:30. The battle goes on between good and evil as believers wrestle with the enemy, rulers, and powers. As Broderson (2004) reminds us, the battle belongs to the Lord (1 Sam 17:47):

> …therefore, we must be strong in the Lord and in the power of his might (Eph 6:10). We have not natural power with which to defeat the forces of darkness. If I am to be victorious, I must draw my strength from the Lord. It was this acknowledgement that gave victory to men like David and Jehoshaphat. (93)

The weapons believers use in this spiritual battle between good and evil are spiritual in nature and are all outlined in the Bible. Jesus modeled the spiritual disciplines including praying alone, reading and meditating on Scripture, and fellowship with others (Matt 6:5; Matt 6:6–7; Luke 11:9; Col 4:2; 1 Thess 5:17). The Lord expects his disciples to read the Word and follow it, "Blessed rather are those who hear the Word of God and obey it" (Luke 11:28). Other ways to fight the battle between good and evil is by serving and giving to the vulnerable (widows, orphans, foreigners, and the poor) using the gifts the Lord has given, fasting and feasting, engaging in times of silence and solitude, weekly Sabbath rest, confession, worship done in spirit and truth, stewardship of the gifts the Lord gives, and life-long learning and growing in faith. Each servant of Christ must be immersed in these spiritual disciplines if they are to be able to fight the good fight and take the gospel to the unreached tribes, tongues, and nations of the world.

Part 4—Culture-Specific Illnesses and Approaches

In medicine and anthropology, culture-specific illnesses, culture-bound syndromes, or folk illnesses can be found discussed in the literature, and are often, but not always localized to a particular cultural group. Many of these patterns of behavior are indigenously considered to be "illnesses," or at least afflictions, and most have local names. Some culture-specific illnesses involve somatic symptoms (pain or disturbed function of a body part), while others are purely behavioral.

According to the American Psychological Association (APA 2022), culture-bound syndromes are a pattern of abnormal behavior that is unique to a specific ethnic or cultural population and does not conform to standard classifications of psychiatric disorders. Culture-bound syndromes differ from region to region, so the reader is encouraged to discover if there are any specific to the area they will be working. APA's perspective is much different than that held by cultural groups who experience these phenomena. According to Ventriglio, et al. (2015):

> Recent changes in the DSM-5 may have abandoned the term "culture-bound syndromes" but in many parts of the world its use continues. Over 60 years ago, these syndromes appeared as exotic, alien, indigenous conditions seen in cultures that were also seen as less psychologically developed. Over the years, many of these syndromes have been reported from multiple cultures using different idioms of distress.
>
> There is no doubt that cultures influence how people experience emotional distress, how they express it and in what terms and, more importantly, from where they seek [medical] help. Historically, colonizers saw those who were being ruled as exotic natives who were perhaps not very psychologically sophisticated and therefore ignorant and objects of observation. These psychiatrists and many anthropologist observers ignored existing indigenous health-care systems, idioms of distress and the therapeutic interventions used by these populations. In many health-care systems, the approach is much more social rather than biological and even when the body is affected, social factors are seen as playing a major role. (3)

When considering the seen and unseen world, and the evidence of continued "cultural illnesses," it is important for believers to understand the social, emotional, and spiritual component of health and illness, and not just the biological and environmental. The quote above presents the idea of indigenous healthcare systems, and systems thinking will be explored more in Lesson 11. When working in cross-cultural contexts, it is essential to not repeat the colonialism mindset of superiority due to perceived differences mentioned in the above quotation. The better method is to use the entry posture discussed before and find out the reasons, causes, and actions of those with different practices and beliefs to learn from and build bridges rather than be judgmental or dismissive.

According to Mianji and Semnani (2015), there is an overlap between spirit possession and cultural syndromes:

> *Zār* refers to a type of spirit, to the illness caused by those spirits who possess humans, and to the rituals needed to pacify those spirits. The zār cult is found throughout northern and eastern African countries such as Sudan, Egypt, Ethiopia, and Somalia, where it is called *sar* as well as some Middle Eastern countries such as Kuwait, Israel, and southern Iran. In these cultures, spirit possession is associated with dissociative episodes such as sudden changes in consciousness or identity that may include periods of shouting, banging of the head against the wall, laughing, singing, or crying. Possessed people may become apathetic or withdrawn or may not be able to accomplish their usual responsibilities. (225)

Many ministry leaders working in areas where demon possession is common are very knowledgeable about the ways to handle these circumstances. Healthcare workers and pastors who go into these cross-cultural experiences who are not familiar with spirit possession and cultural syndromes can look to the local leaders for guidance.

Learning Activities

- **Read** "Zār Spirit Possession in Iran and African Countries" (Mianji & Semnani, https://bit.ly/3u9lHWt) to understand more about a medical and secular perspective of spirit possession and cultural bound syndromes seen in different places around the world. Compare the medical and secular view to a biblical view of caring for people wholistically: showing love, care, and compassion for the whole person as a fellow image bearer of God and one in need of the liberating power of the gospel of Jesus Christ.

- **Read** "Cultural Differences and the Communication of the Gospel" (Paul Hiebert, https://bit.ly/3U86Vdg) as a helpful reminder of cultural differences that have been presented in the past few lessons and ways to more effectively share the gospel message across different dimensions of culture.

Regions around the world have different healthcare and spiritual practices they may use. Review a few of them on the internet, and if there is one you know of that is not listed, add it to the list for discussion with the group during the weekly zoom meeting.

Traditional Practices (chart)

Practice	Country/Region Practiced	What does it entail?
Ayurveda		
Siddha Medicine		
Unani		
Yin and Yang		
Cupping		
Coining		
Muti		
Ifa		
Voodoo		
Other Practices?		

References

Broderson, B. (2004). *Spiritual Warfare: Fighting the Good Fight of Faith*. Back to Basics Publishing.

Cozens, S. (2018). "Cultures, Fear Cultures, and Guilt Cultures: Reviewing the Evidence." *International Bulletin of Mission Research*. DOI:10.1177/2396939318764087.

Elmer, D. (2002). *Cross-cultural Connections: Stepping Out and Fitting In around the World*. Downers Grove, IL: InterVarsity Press.

Elmer, D. (2006). *Cross-cultural Servanthood: Serving the World in Christlike Humility*. Downers Grove, IL: InterVarsity Press.

Fountain, D. (1989). *Health, the Bible, and the Church*. Billy Graham Center: Biblical Perspectives on Health and Healing.

Galanti, G. (2015). *Caring for Patients from Different Cultures* (5th ed.). Philadelphia, PA: University of Pennsylvania Press.

Hollister, S. (2018). Placenta Burial Rituals. https://placentarisks.org/wp-content/uploads/2018/09/Placenta-burial-rituals-from-around-the-world-handout.pdf.

Lucenay, N. (2019). *How to Recognize Different Cultures: Guilt, Shame, and Fear*. Beyond the Front Door: Cultural Differences Blog, https://nancylucenay.com/how-to-recognize-different-cultures-guilt-shame-and-fear/.

Mianji, F., and Semnani, Y. (2015). "Zār Spirit Possession in Iran and African Countries: Group Distress, Culture-bound Syndrome or Cultural Concept of Distress?" *Iran Journal of Psychiatry*, 10 (4): 225–32.

Myers, B. (2011). *Walking with the Poor: Principles and Practices of Transformational Development*. New York, NY: Orbis Books.

Nida, E. (1954). *Customs and Cultures: Anthropology for Christian Missions*. New York, NY: Harper and Brothers.

Pratt, Z., Sills, D., and Walters, J. (2014). *Introduction to Global Missions*. Nashville, TN: B and H Publishing Group.

Richardson, D. (2005). *The Peace Child: An Unforgettable Story of Primitive Jungle Treachery in the 20th Century*. Ventura, CA: Regal Books.

Ventriglio, A., Ayonrinde, O., and Bhugra, D. (2015). "Relevance of Culture-bound Syndromes in the 21st Century." *Psychiatry and Clinical Neurosciences*. DOI:10.1111/pcn.12359.

Reflection Questions for Group Discussion

1. What did you learn about the excluded middle you did not know before reading this lesson?

2. How do guilt, shame, and fear as they relate to the biblical concept of sin manifest in cultures around the world?

3. List ways the enemy may cause doubt and seek to destroy a cross-cultural ministry.

4. Describe criteria you would use to discern which folk medicine practices can be embraced?

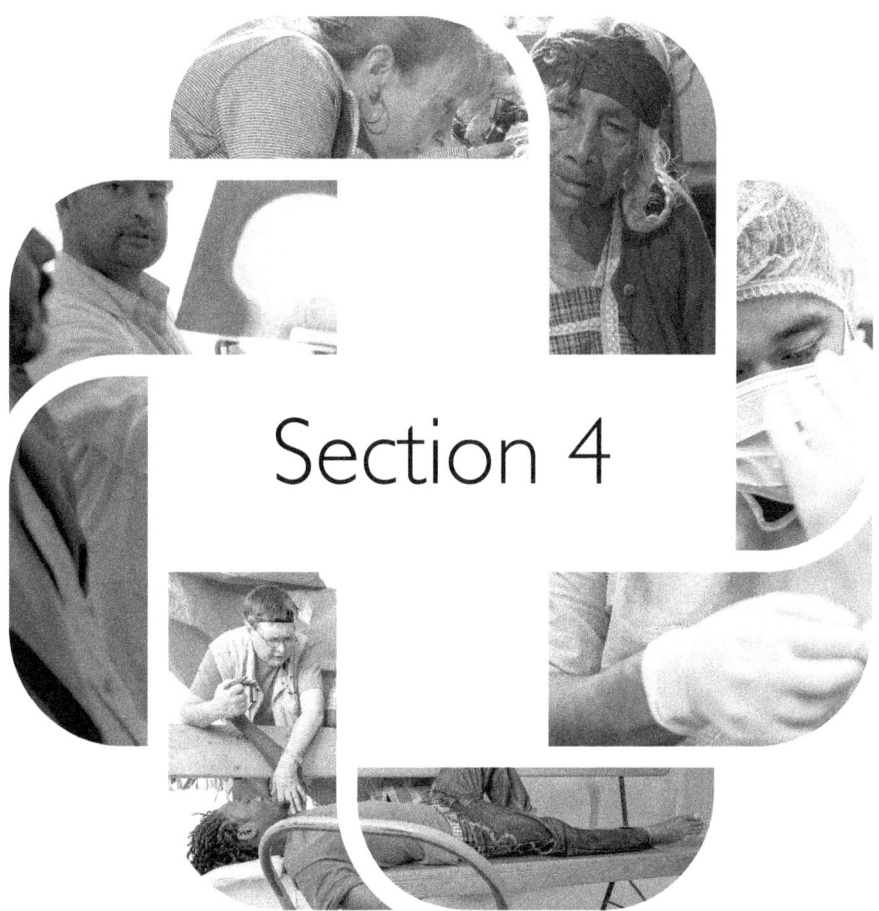

Section 4

Strategic Innovation

Arnold Gorske and Rebecca Meyer (Lesson 10)
Perry Jansen and Rebecca Meyer (Lesson 11)
Mike Soderling and Rebecca Meyer (Lesson 12)

Lesson 10
Health Promotion and Disease Prevention

Summary	Knowledge Objectives
Building on the previous 3 sections, this lesson describes the health-promoting and disease preventing (HPandP) responsibility of every Christian and every church. and provides examples of how biblically inspired wholistic global transformation and healing can be accomplished in community.	1. Explain why Christian missionaries developed HPandP and the Primary Care System. 2. Recognize the critical importance of the participatory approach to resolution of healthcare problems at all levels of care including direction from and collaboration with the local community as well as the Ministry of Health and local healthcare providers.
Thematic Content	**Attitude Objectives**
• Biblically inspired, evidence-based HPandP systems were developed by Christian missionaries and strongly endorsed by the WHO to this day. • Faith and evidence are keys to promoting heath, especially through Primary Health Care • Evidence-based international standards and guidelines (ISandGs) are important to follow for saving the most lives and preventing the most suffering. • Biblically based approaches promote global health and well-being, and Jesus's methods of teaching, touching, and restoring relationships is the way to grow the kingdom. • Wholistic Health models create a framework to promote health for all and grow the kingdom in all the world.	1. Relate the hazards of attempting to utilize the wrong approach in a Short-Term Mission strategy. 2. Describe the evidence-based importance of following the healing example of Jesus. 3. Describe how simple congregation-based health promotion and disease prevention can help resolve 70% of the disease burden that is preventable.
Conceptual Thread—Health Promotion	**Practice (Skills) Objectives**
Health promotion is a way to engage and empower individuals and communities to choose healthy behaviors and make changes that reduce the risk of developing chronic diseases and other morbidities. Defined by the World Health Organization, health promotion enables people to increase control over their own health.	1. (Long term) Design a church-based health promotion and disease prevention program with your pastor and church council (or FBO board) for your community's health. 2. Using freely available biblical and evidence-based resources, implement an empowering educational system for pressing community health needs. 3. Explain to your pastor and church council (or FBO board) how a church-based health fair can promote Jesus's model of health and healing as well as "grow the church."

Part 1—Health Promotion

"When Christ commissioned his disciples to heal, he was not addressing the graduating class of a healing profession. He was laying an obligation on *all* who would follow him" (McGilvray 1981, 51).

Christianity is by far the largest religious group in the world, and in 2020 there are about 2.518 billion members. Yet there is much to be done and places the church does not exist. How can health promotion and disease prevention (HPandP) be utilized to enable *each* of these members to not only meet their biblical health and healing responsibilities as stewards of their own bodies and natural resources, but to demonstrate Christ's love effectively and powerfully to their communities and beyond?

How would this impact our most important local and global health care crises, including potentially disastrous future pandemics? How would meeting this responsibility for our neighbor affect global health? And how does all this grow the kingdom of God in every nation?

> Heal the sick who are there and tell them,
> the kingdom of God has come near to you. (Luke 10:9)

> All authority in heaven and on earth has been given to me.
> Therefore, go and make disciples of all nations, baptizing them
> in the name of the Father and of the Son and of the Holy Spirit,
> and teaching them to obey everything I have commanded you.
> And surely, I am with you always, to the very end of the age.
> (Matt 28:19–20)

> One of the most urgent needs of today is that Christian congregations, in collaboration with Christian medical workers, should again recognise and exercise the healing ministry which belongs properly to them.
> (McGilvray 1981, 34)

Health Promotion and Disease Prevention (HPandP) in Primary Health Care—the Critical History of Public Health Care and Modern-Day Need for HPandP

In the 1960's studies from the World Council of Churches had documented that the church's hospital-based curative care health system was expensive, inefficient, and non-sustainable. To address these critical deficiencies, the Christian Medical Commission (CMC) in the 1960s developed a more wholistic health promotion and disease prevention-based system as the foundation of what they called Primary Health Care (PHC), a whole-of-society approach that includes health promotion, disease prevention, treatment, rehabilitation, and palliative care. This system was based on a mission objective of *shalom* and Jesus's contextualized whole person, team-based ministry. It was incorporated into WHO's 1978 *Declaration of Alma Ata*, co-authored by Carl Taylor, a Christian missionary member of the CMC, as an efficient and effective way to achieve health for all.

WHO's 2008 World Health Report, *Primary Care—Now More than Ever*, emphasized the following as one of the most critical problems in both developed and developing countries: "Misdirected care: Resource allocation clusters around curative services at great cost, neglecting the potential of *primary prevention and health promotion* to prevent up to *70% of the disease burden.*"

WHO's 2018 *Declaration of Astana* reaffirmed "the commitments expressed in the ambitious and visionary Declaration of Alma Ata of 1978 …We can no longer underemphasize the crucial importance of *health promotion and disease prevention, nor tolerate fragmented, unsafe or poor-quality care*…We will prioritize *disease prevention and health promotion* and will aim to meet all people's health needs across the life course…All people, countries and organizations are encouraged to support this movement." Although the community-based PHC approach (vs a market-driven fragmented curative care approach) was not adequately or only slowly implemented as hoped in many countries, including in the US, it remains the foundation of WHO's current approach to global health.

Although originally intended as a ministry of the congregation, HPandP has now become the foundation for the rapidly growing secular field of Lifestyle Medicine. This has greatly expanded the evidence-base not only for prevention of our most important non-communicable diseases (NCDs), but for prevention of communicable diseases, and wholistic, first-line treatment of many conditions cared for in primary care.

HPandP Approaches Enable Congregations to Assume their Role as a Provider of Health and Healing to the Community

Curative care-focused health systems result in multiple times the cost per person and yet perform poorly in health metrics compared to countries which follow HPandP-based PHC guidelines (e.g. US is now 43rd below others in outcomes). Therefore, churches' HPandP services *to their own* communities are therefore critically needed. These preventive and promotive services are possible even in low resource settings.

However, attempting to provide congregation-based curative care is especially complex and potentially dangerous, especially through short-term endeavors. For example, despite its pharmacovigilance safeguards, adverse drug reactions in US hospitals are the *4th leading cause of death*. NSAIDs in arthritis patients in the US alone cause 16,500 deaths/year due to gastrointestinal complications. As documented by numerous *Best Practices in Global Health Missions* (BPGHM, *Short-term Health Missions—Quality of Care*) there are risks for patients treated with a drug-based curative care approach on short-term missions (STMs) when no or limited local curative care services are available to manage potentially serious adverse drug reactions or surgical complications. That is why it is important for short-term groups to recognize and even partner with those long-term endeavors of mission agencies who have sent nurses and doctors to learn the language, culture, and provide compassionate clinical care.

Evidence-based curative care remains essential in faith-based organizations, (FBO) hospitals and clinics which can provide pharmacovigilance and other safety, quality monitoring, and follow-up systems in place to mitigate harm. These can meet critical gaps in service, especially in remote areas or disasters. When coupled with HPandP services and collaboration with the local churches, and in conjunction with long-term public health measures such as food access, building latrines and clean water sources to prevent ongoing infection, the community impact can be tremendous. Working closely with existing local FBO clinics or hospitals, the Ministry of Health, or local healthcare providers expand the mission of each.

Although most congregations throughout the world do not have the material and professional resources to provide safe and effective curative care, *all* congregations have the human assets and leadership to follow Jesus's commands to teach all the life-promoting ways which lead to human flourishing, preventing 70% of the disease burden in their communities. Examples of how the congregation can meet its health and healing responsibilities through HPandP include the following (See BPGHM *Church and Healthcare* for numerous additional examples).

The 12 Principles of Kingdom Healthcare (Carolyn Klaus 2019)

1. It must be available to all, especially the poor
2. It turns no one away, but it need not be free
3. It empowers people to obtain health for themselves
4. It focuses on prevention, both for the individual and the community
5. It is wholistic, bringing people into physical, mental, emotional, social, spiritual, and economic health
6. It is a ministry of the church
7. It must be excellent
8. It must be rooted in prayer
9. It must demonstrate the supernatural
10. It respects God as the giver and taker of life
11. It occasionally confronts the system
12. Its staff must be servants of God
13. List Others:

Learning Activities

- **Watch**—CCIH Webinar "Healing and the Church: What Is Our Calling?" from 13:00 to 37:00 including "12 Principles of Kingdom Healthcare" (https://bit.ly/3Ont83n).
- **Read**—Seager, Seager, and Tazelaar, "The Perils and Promise of Short-Term Healthcare Missions" (https://bit.ly/4bdNCoU).

Reflection Questions

1. How does a diverse, team-based approach lead to wholistic healing?
2. How can you apply Dr. Klaus' 12 Principles of Kingdom Healthcare on the local and global level?
3. What steps can you take to redeem the shortcomings of short-term healthcare missions?

Part 2—Faith as a Key to the Success of Primary Healthcare

Congregation-based HPandP in collaboration with the local community, local healthcare systems, and the ministry of health remains the key to meeting the WHO primary health care vision, and for the promotion of *shalom* and transformational development —CMC's vision of health and wholeness for all. The UN's Social Determinants of Health (https://sdgs.un.org/goals) play an important role in the health of individuals, families, and communities. They may be biological, behavioral, socioeconomic, psychosocial, or social. They include some of the following areas:

1. Social and physical environment
2. Genetics and biology
3. Income level and poverty
4. Educational opportunities

5. Occupation, employment status, and workplace safety
6. Gender inequity
7. Ethnic and racial segregation
8. Food insecurity, food deserts, and inaccessibility of nutritious food choices
9. Access to housing and utility services
10. Early childhood experiences and development
11. Social support and community inclusivity
12. Crime rates and exposure to violent behavior
13. Availability of transportation
14. Neighborhood conditions and physical environment
15. Access to safe drinking water, clean air, and toxin-free environments
16. Recreational and leisure opportunities

From NEJM https://catalyst.nejm.org/doi/full/10.1056/CAT.17.0312.

However, these secular efforts leave enormous gaps due to their inability (or unwillingness) to address the underlying spiritual, moral, religious, and behavioral elements. There is only recent scholarly interest in religion and spirituality as a key social determinant of health (Idler 2014; Oman 2018).

The WHO recognizes the high value of faith and local faith communities for global health. *Building from Common Foundations* (WHO 2008) confirms the critical role of the congregation and emphasizes the numerous assets local congregations already have available to provide these services, and to teach health-promoting behaviors. More importantly, the Scriptures paint a clear picture of restored *shalom* and should be our overarching motivation. The Word provides a depth of wisdom guiding the believer to spread the gospel and provide excellent care.

Part 3—Transformational Development and Community Health Evangelism/Education

Transformational Development is an approach that leads to sustainable well-being. The Community Health Evangelism/Education (CHE) strategy developed by Stan Rowland is based on community development, local ownership, integration (wholism), and gospel multiplication. It utilizes local resources, participatory approaches to problem solving, Bible learning, prayer, and servant leadership, and is being deployed around the world to enhance the physical, social, and biblical health of communities and urban neighborhoods. Community Health Workers are community members called and dedicated to promoting health in their communities and are thought to be the key to health for all, trained and empowered by health professionals to offer more widespread services.

Learning Activities

- **Read**—The WHO's "Building from Common Foundations," Executive Summary and Introduction, 5–6, and Ways Forward 27–29 (https://bit.ly/3OjOdM4).
- **Read**—Kiser, Jones, and Gunderson, "Faith and Health: Leadership Aligning Assets to Transform Communities" (https://bit.ly/3Ui8Dst).

Questions—Participatory Approach, CHE, and Assets

- **Read**—"CHE Core Values" (https://bit.ly/3Hz26SP).
- **Watch**—CHE "Neighborhood Transformation" (https://bit.ly/3UjSx1B).
- **Watch**—LIA's "Life in Abundance Model" video (https://vimeo.com/133020033).

After watching the videos about transformational development and CHE, answer the questions below. Be prepared to discuss your thoughts with the group.

1. How do you think a participatory approach contributes to community ownership and sustainability?

2. Why do you think this Community Health Education/Evangelism approach to development is now being adopted by US secular organizations for facilitating behavior change in "lifestyle medicine"?

3. Choose two of the Health Education Participatory Lesson Plans from the CHE Network list (https://bit.ly/3x2zFur) and describe how these could change behavior toward better health.

4. List 10 religious health assets which are available through you and your congregation.

Part 4—Utilizing Biblical Evidence for Principles and Practices

Section 1 of this course gave a biblical framework upon which to build a strategy for health in mission. The authority of international standards and guidelines must be interpreted in the light of the authority of the revealed Word of God. YHWH's desire to dwell with his people, to respond to their pain, to set them free from captivity, to expose and drive out the corrupting and disease-resulting effects of sin, and to create a community of health and life in the land is our pattern. Jesus's loving incarnation, healing touch, transformative teaching, atoning death, hopeful resurrection, and ongoing presence in his people from every tribe, tongue and nation is an expression of God's desire and our supreme model.

Jesus Healed Through Touch, Faith, Teaching, and Through the Human Body

> I have often wondered why Jesus so frequently (the Bible records *nearly always*) touched the people he healed…With his power he easily could…raising his hands to heal *en masse*…He wanted those people, one by one, to feel his love and warmth and his full identification with them. Jesus knew he could not readily demonstrate love to a crowd, for love usually involves touching. (Yancy and Brand 1997, 138–40)

"Daughter, your faith has healed you" (Luke 8:48). "Rise and go, your faith has made you whole" (Luke 17:19). Numerous WHO reports and WHO "Quality of Life Assessments" also recognize the importance of the spiritual aspects of health. And reports from the US National Institutes of Health document how our "beliefs and values initiate a neurohormonal cascade that results in the healing response." This is evidenced in the medical sciences. Spiritual beliefs, lifestyle and prayer can be very important for healing of individuals and communities. He used healing moments to teach deep spiritual, social, emotional, and environmental truths. The Sermon on the Mount occurred on the heels of healing all who came to him which elicited large crowds, "and he began to teach them" (Matt 4:23–5:2).

> We in medicine need to restore our patient's confidence in the most powerful healer in the world: the human body … The mind, not the cells of the injured (part) will determine the final extent of rehabilitation … Doctors tend to exaggerate their own significance in the scheme of things … A human being, unlike any machine, contains what Schweitzer called "the doctor within" the ability to repair itself and to affect consciously the healing process." (Brand 1993)

From a biblical as well as scientific evidence-based standpoint perhaps the most important truth in all of healthcare is this: Our bodies were designed to be self-healing and to respond to our beliefs—and God is our healer and sustainer. He cares about our embodied life. Jesus, through both teaching and example, emphasized this 2000 years before either the NIH or the WHO measured its importance. The majority of the healing effect of many of our most commonly used medications is primarily due to this "Faith" or "Placebo" effect.

Part 5—Wholistic Health Models

There have been several health paradigms that have shifted over time among global health leaders. In the twentieth century these included the Hospital-based Pathogenic Biomedical Paradigm, the Community-based Bio-Sanitary Pathogenic Paradigm, the Health-genic Systemic Ecological Paradigm of Comprehensive Health (see DeAngulo and Losada 2015).

To participate in any effective healing paradigm will require positioning oneself in the broader scope of God's communal activity in redeeming the world. Finding a comprehensive wholistic model for transformational development is an important goal as each takes his or her unique position, being a prophetic voice, which influences and critiques international standards, enhancing them, and informing them.

This would include trust-building, caring concern, and faithfulness at the point of individual care. Health promotion and disease prevention are empowered by biblically informed directives, including promoting virtues such as temperance, discipline, eschewing pleasures, relational harmony, sexual integrity, body stewardship, prayer for healing, meditation (on the Word of God), deferred gratification, truth-speaking in love (Eph 4:15; 1 John 3:18), eschewing vice (sin), communal thinking (loving neighbor), etc.

Church-based health fairs are relatively inexpensive and mobilize church member nurses or other healthcare providers as well as other volunteers to provide HPandP-based screening, monitoring, prayer, counselling, health education, and timely referral to professional health services. Missionary doctors like Drs Brand, Fountain, Burkitt, and Trowell have long emphasized the critical importance of personal lifestyle in promoting biblically based solutions to our most important diseases and world problems. Their pleas were wise because they spoke as physicians well informed by caring for patients in need. Unfortunately, their wisdom has gone largely unheeded, and we now face not only the 3 WHO "Slow Motion Disasters" of non-communicable diseases (NCDs), climate change, and antimicrobial resistance. Many of these could have been prevented had the global community simply responded to their pleas years ago.

Following Christ: Ten Marks of Christ-Centered Ministry	
Servant Leadership	• Submission to the Father. • Filled, Led, and Empowered by the Holy Spirit.
Faithfulness-Focused Strategies	• Prayerful Strategic Planning. • Raising Kingdom Resources.
Eternity-Oriented Metrics	• Ministry Accountability. • Transparent Financial Administration.
Relationship-Based Management	• Serving People Humbly. • Doing Everything with Love.
Stewardship View of Resources	• Mobilizing Spiritually Gifted People. • Radical Christian Generosity.

Adapted from Hoag, G., Rodin, S., and Wilmer, W. (2014). *The choice: Christ-centered pursuit of kingdom outcomes.* ECFA Press, 53.

Learning Activities

- **Read**—DeAngulo, Jose Miguel, Losada, Luz Stella. "Health Paradigm Shifts in the 20th Century." *Christian Journal for Global Health* 2(1), 2015: 49–58 (bit.ly/48iPtG8).

- **Review**—box above.

- **Reflect**—Which historical modern-day Paradigms of Health are most compelling? Write down four ways a person could use this information to improve health outcomes and kingdom impact.

References

DeAngulo, Jose Miguel, Losada, Luz Stella. "Health Paradigm Shifts in the 20th Century." *Christian Journal for Global Health* 2(1), 2015: 49–58. https://doi.org/10.15566/cjgh.v2i1.37.

Global CHE Network. https://www.chenetwork.org/.

Hoag, G., Rodin, S., and Wilmer, W. (2014). *The Choice: Christ-centered Pursuit of Kingdom Outcomes.* ECFA Press.

Idler, E. (2014). *Religion as a Social Determinant of Public Health.* New York: Oxford University Press.

Kiser, M. Jones, D. L., and Gunderson, G. R. (2006). "Faith and Health: Leadership Aligning Assets to Transform Communities." *International Review of Mission* 95: 376–77.

Magezi, Vhumani. "Church-driven Primary Health Care: Models for an Integrated Church and Community Primary Health Care in Africa (a case study of the Salvation Army in East Africa)." *HTS Teologiese Studies/ Theological Studies* 74(2): 4365. https://doi.org/10.4102/hts.v74i2.4365.

McGilvray, J. (1981). *The Quest for Health and Wholeness.* Tubingen: German Institute for Medical Missions.

Oman, D. (2018). *Why Religion and Spirituality Matter for Public Health—Evidence, Implications, and Resources.* Springer.

Seager, G., Seager, C., and Tazelaar, G. (2010). "The Perils and Promise of Short-term Healthcare Missions." *Journal of Christian Nursing* 27(3): 262–66. https://doi.org/10.1097/CNJ.0b013e3181e06f33.

Social Determinants of Health (2017). *NEJM Catalyst* https://catalyst.nejm.org/doi/full/10.1056/CAT.17.0312.

United Nations UN. (2021). Environmental and Social Determinants of Health.

World Health Organization, WHO. (1978). *Health for All by the Year 2000.* Alma Ata Declaration. https://www.who.int/.

World Health Organization, WHO. (2008). *Building from Common Foundations: The World Health Organization and Faith-Based Organizations in Primary Healthcare.* Geneva Global Performance Philanthropy.

Yancy, P., and Brand, P. (1997). *Fearfully and Wonderfully Made.* Zondervan.

Reflection Questions for Group Discussion

After completing the lesson answer the following questions. Be prepared to participate in a facilitated discussion afterward.

1. How can a Christian promote health and prevent disease within their context related to common health problems such as obesity, smoking, diabetes, and hypertension?

2. How do you think a participatory approach contributes to community ownership and sustainability of health promotion strategies?

3. Why do you think a Community Health Education/Evangelism approach to development is now being adopted by US secular organizations for facilitating behavior change in "lifestyle medicine"?

4. List 5 religious health assets (resources) which are available through you and your congregation.

Lesson 11
Churches, Hospitals, and Health Systems

Summary	Knowledge Objectives
Health-related missions have continually undergone transformation and evolution in response to new knowledge, technologies, and socio-political realities. Like all other "complex systems," there are many factors that influence the impact of healthcare missions. This section "unpacks" some of the trends and tensions that exist within modern healthcare missions.	1. Review the use of community-based and church-based health ministry domestically and internationally. 2. Review the history and impact of mission hospitals and health ministries of national churches. 3. Discuss how disease and population are interrelated and create challenges and opportunities for healthcare missions focus. 4. Discuss the ways assessment and outcome measurement are important in healthcare strategies, as well as their limitations.
Thematic Content	**Attitude Objectives**
• Exploring the multiple models and strategies for healthcare mission. • Considering the shifting paradigms of health and healthcare missions. • Appreciating the distinction and role of the church, the hospital, and the health system in healthcare mission. • Identifying the key gaps where healthcare mission is vital. • The emerging science and tools of Systems Thinking and its application to healthcare mission. • Consider how we measure and improve our impact.	1. Appreciate the difference between a linear, cause-and-effect understanding of health systems and a complex adaptive system approach. 2. Understand who could or should be included in asset-based and/or collaborative approaches. 3. Appreciate the potential for disparities in resources (material, social, and spiritual) amongst unreached peoples.
Conceptual Thread—Contextualization	**Practice (Skills) Objectives**
Contextualization is the process and practice of expressing the gospel and living out the life of the church in a new cultural context. Biblical understanding considers the context of the biblical writers and is then applied to various global cultural and language contexts but does not compromise the essential truths of the gospel truth.	1. Anticipate future trends in disease prevalence and populations using epidemiologic data. 2. Map out distinctions, systems, relationships, and perspectives in key problems faced personally, professionally, or in ministry. 3. Design and implement meaningful metrics for the impact of healthcare mission activities.

Part 1—Strategies and Models in Global Health Mission

The lessons in prior sections have summarized how "medical missions" has evolved over the centuries since Christ first modeled wholistic care. This evolution has been influenced by geopolitical events, theological and philosophical shifts, the advent of modern transportation and communication, and advances in medicine. The shifts have uncovered new opportunities for advancing spiritual objectives (salvation, church planting and growth), social objectives (justice, peace) and physical objectives (improved health, ecology, and healthcare). As we consider the current state of global health missions, there are remnants of old models that remain, and some that are still quite relevant. In contrast, others may have become barriers to accomplishing these larger objectives.

The term "medical missions" will have different meanings depending upon who you are and what you've experienced (refer back to earlier content in Lessons 4–6). For some, "mission" means "someone from **here** going over **there** to help the poor and unevangelized." We have explored the history of the mission hospitals bringing modern advances in western medicine together with the Good News of Jesus Christ.

The term "mission" may imply a primary focus on evangelism, conversion, and church planting. This course emphasizes that the provision of healthcare should not be seen as merely a "means" to the higher "end" of personal salvation and the establishment of a church but something more integral to living out the kingdom of God. The practice of healthcare (including public health) is a calling by God to use our skills for his service wherever possible. The result is the multi-faceted nature of global health missions reflecting multiple opportunities, perspectives, and callings.

Learning Activities

- **Fill-in**—"SWOT Analysis" (strategies worksheet below*).* SWOT analysis is a helpful tool used across industries and businesses, including healthcare, as an assessment to measure strengths, weaknesses, opportunities, and threats within an organization, or before beginning a new plan/activity.

- **Reflect**—The "SWOT Analysis" lists several models or strategies still playing an important role in healthcare mission.

    i. Consider each model and its brief description.

    ii. In the spaces provided, first consider the strengths of each model.

    iii. What needs is it able to meet?

    iv. How does it contribute to the health of the community?

    v. How does it reflect what Christ is calling the church to?

    vi. How does it honor the culture and values of the community?

    vii. How does it build capacity within the church, community, and nation?

Strategies in Medical Missions SWOT Analysis	Strengths and Opportunities	Threats/Hazards and Weaknesses
Short-Term Mission Trips Teams of medical providers sent to provide healthcare services in a foreign country or region, usually in partnership with a local church, ministry, or health facility.		
Mission Hospitals Permanent hospital facilities in target countries. Often historically founded by western missionaries. May have planted churches and denominations who have varying degrees of ownership/control over hospital operations. Often integrated into national health system.		
Community Health Programs Usually based in poor, rural communities with a strong emphasis on prevention and primary healthcare (routine child health and maternity services). May integrate church planting or be integrated as a ministry of the local church. Often with only basic "curative" services (malaria, diarrhea).		
Disaster Response Teams Teams of medical and logistics personnel who respond to a natural disaster or other emergency (i.e., conflict, displaced persons camps) to provide routine and emergency medical services. Often includes provision of shelter, food, basic healthcare, basic education.		
Domestic Healthcare Clinics Faith-based community clinics that target underserved areas for routine and basic curative services. Often function as important safety-net providers for their communities. Sometimes connected with a local church and have varying levels of spiritual care integration. Some operate as free clinics, relying on fundraising from donors. Others may receive government funds through public programs.		
Creative access/Marketplace workers Mission-minded health personnel who take jobs in settings that might be closed to formal "missionaries," but welcome western-trained medical providers and medical educators. Freedom to openly evangelize may be very limited by the laws of the country or culture.		

1. As you considered the various healthcare mission strategies outlined in the SWOT analysis, which strategy were you most familiar with?
2. Which strategy do you think best reflects your passion for healthcare mission?

Part 2—What Is the Role of the Church in Healthcare?

We have explored the Christian faith and the church's role in responding to human needs, suffering, and disease. Behind each medical mission movement were Christian philanthropists and churches preparing and sending missionaries. Most missionary efforts aimed to reach the lost with the good news of the gospel toward personal salvation and the establishing a healthy and replicating national church. The provision of public health, primary healthcare and curative health services is not merely a means to an end but is part and parcel of bringing *shalom* to a community and reflecting the kingdom of God.

The provision of preventative health, primary health care, and curative care as a direct function of the church has been partially accomplished in some developing countries as a maturation of "mission" hospitals to "church" hospitals. In some cases, church leadership mistakenly sees the hospital as an income generator for the church rather than a conduit for the church's ministry to the community. However, often the entities of church and hospital function independently. In more developed countries, these linkages are only historical. A deeper understanding of the spiritual nature of disease would help believers worldwide address spiritual issues, social and physical consequences of sin, and the power of "right relationship" (*shalom*) to bring health.

The Christian church, if seen as a whole, represents one of the largest, most respected, and most diverse organizations on earth. Most governments and multilateral organizations (UN and World Bank) recognize the critical role faith-based organizations (FBOs), faith leaders, and faith itself play in health and development. In sub-Saharan Africa, faith-based church hospitals provide up to 40% of health services. Current movements toward universal health coverage and improvements in maternal-child health will also require engagement with the church and church-based hospitals and clinics.

Churches and Communities—Domestic Healthcare Mission and Health Inequities

Many churches recognize their responsibility to meet their communities' physical, social, and spiritual needs. Church programs take many shapes and sizes, from housing food banks to providing childcare to free medical and dental clinics. For example, the Christian Community Health Fellowship (www.cchf.org) is a network of health centers that continue to provide free or publicly funded health services for underserved and uninsured members of their communities in the US. These clinics serve as safety nets for millions of people who could not otherwise access health services. Many of these organizations also have programs or links to programs that provide social services such as counseling, housing assistance, nutrition programs, and community development.

The disparities in health outcomes and access to health services across the globe have resulted from a long history of inequities and systemic injustices that have denied some citizens (especially communities of color) access to an environment that promotes health. Similarly, health outcome disparities between countries are due to complex historical, political, economic, and environmental factors that have resulted in deep inequities for specific populations. Understanding the historical roots of these inequities is vital to help address the social and political change required to begin reversing them.

The church can play a role in addressing not only the health needs of its population but also the more profound societal failures that contribute to poverty, corruption, injustice, and discrimination. Demonstrating Christ's love in word and deed requires acknowledging the biblical realities of sin, redemption, salvation, discipleship, and sanctification.

Churches, Hospitals, and Health Systems

Learning Activities
- **Watch**—"Equity vs. Equality" (https://bit.ly/3vZfhts).
- **Reflect**—Write down several differences between "equality" and "equity" in healthcare access.
- **For Supplemental Reading**—Cochrane & Gunderson, "People Who Congregate: Building on Strengths" (https://bit.ly/47Vc0c5).

Part 3—Community-Based Health Interventions

The community and its institutions play enormous roles in the health of its citizens, especially in health promotion and disease prevention (HPandP). Apart from people groups where the church has not yet been planted, the church is a vital part of the community in most low- and middle-income countries. However, most see public health and prevention programs as the responsibility of "the state" (the country's government). Most governments do not have the resources or political will to implement a complete package of public health measures or deliver sufficient healthcare services. Churches and hospital leadership often have strong relationships with the communities they serve, and are "trusted" partners, even in places where Christians are a small minority.

When developing public health and primary healthcare services, it is critical to involve the community in planning and prioritizing care. When the community and its beneficiaries participate in developing their own solutions, implementation is more likely, and there is greater ownership and long-term sustainability. Community engagement in health can also be a powerful ministry for evangelism and discipleship. Programs like Community Health Evangelism/ Education (CHE) have developed Christ-centered community development curricula and programs that integrate discipleship and health promotion (https://chenetwork.org).

Disaster Response and Complex Health Emergencies

Natural disasters, violent conflicts, and displaced populations are an increasing problem. They rapidly place thousands of people at risk for devastating health and social consequences. These crises create opportunities for the Body of Christ to respond to suffering and insecurity when people are in greatest need. Indeed, several Christian organizations consistently and competently react to these natural and man-made crises in a way that genuinely reflects Christ and the gospel.

A significant proportion of the funds for disaster response comes from their close international relationships with churches and individual believers. Because these target populations are especially vulnerable, responders must be sensitive to how care and support are provided so that it does not cause further harm to people already experiencing trauma and insecurity.

The Sphere Handbook has useful guidelines and tools that can assist organizations in developing appropriate responses to complex humanitarian crises (bit.ly/3I2aQ4c).

Learning Activities
- **Review**—Core Humanitarian Standards (see figure on the next page).
- **Reflect**—Critique the 4 Sphere principles in light of Scripture—humanity, impartiality, independence, and neutrality and the 9 Core Humanitarian Standards depicted in the figure.

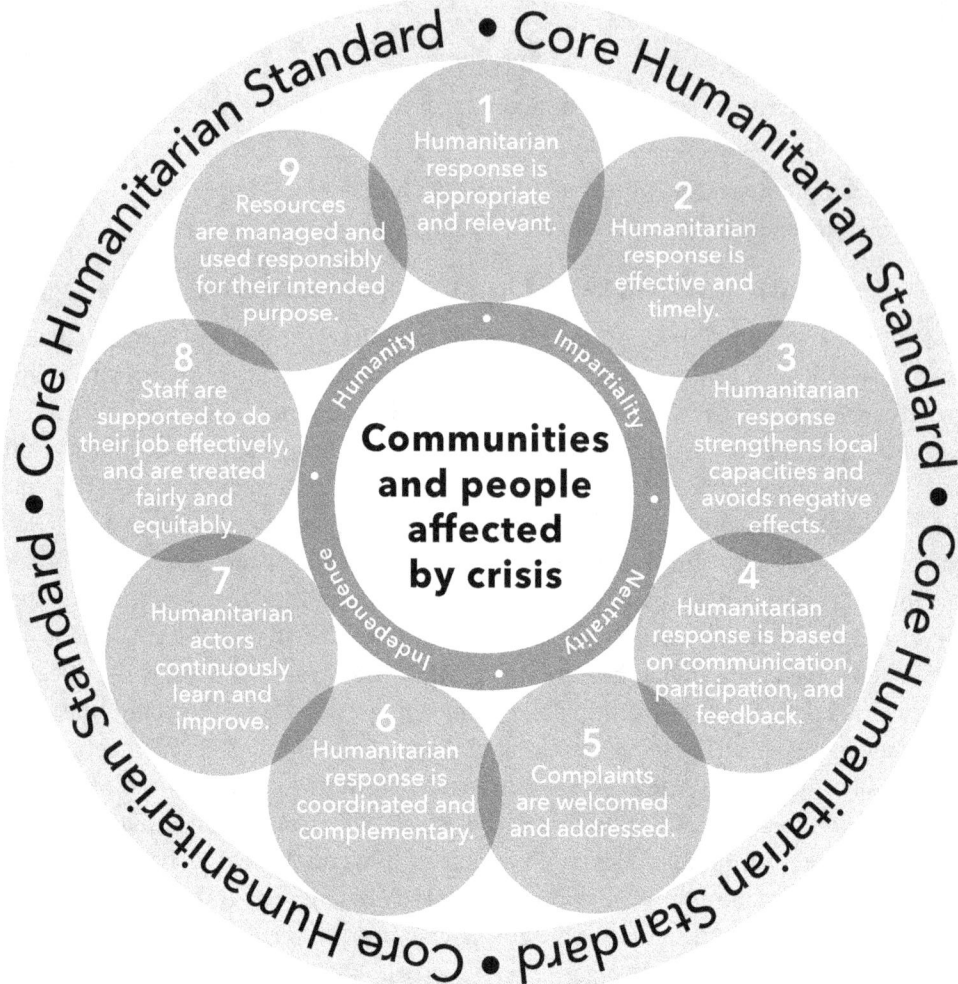

Figure 8: Nine Core Humanitarian Standards

Part 4—Mission Hospitals to Indigenous, Christ-centered, Whole-Person Care

Healthcare missions, evangelism, and discipleship go hand-in-hand—they are all necessary components of wholistic outreach. As a church is being established, it is essential to identify and engage the gifts, talents, and callings of individual church members as part of the greater goals of the congregation. Mentoring, training, and discipleship occur as leaders are identified from within. Leaders and members train others while learning and growing in their faith. As the church becomes stronger, the members learn how to care for the physical, social, and spiritual needs of church members as well as their community and beyond. In this way, the whole church body develops an understanding of its wholistic role in the Great Commission.

The development of healthcare ministry needs to be just as deliberate a process as building church leadership and capacity. Developing national healthcare leadership should be a major benchmark for successful healthcare mission.

Serving the healthcare needs of the poor will always require resources from those with more resources. Thoughtful "inter-dependence" between the "sending" church and the "receiving" church requires great humility and trusting relationships. Foreign missionaries generally serve at no cost to the local church or mission hospital and often are better able to access financial and other resources. This contributes to an imbalance of power and the potential for poor alignment of priorities. Application of systems thinking, exploring healthy cross-cultural partnerships, and identifying a shared vision, mission and goals are critical to the long-term success of mission hospitals and health programs.

The ideal long-term goal of any mission hospital should be to see a healthy, locally "owned," Christ-centered healthcare ministry that focuses on whole-person care (physical, social, psychological, and spiritual). This should include a strategy for caring for the poor and vulnerable in the community. As the local church matures, these ministries will "own" their biblical call to "send" people and resources to minister to those outside their community. This transition often takes decades, if not generations, but if it is not explicitly a part of the ministry's strategy, it will never happen.

Learning Activities

- **Read**—Jansen, P. "Health Systems Strengthening Through the Faith-Based Sector in India" (Results: Themes section 107–11) (https://bit.ly/3OjuXOG).

- **Reflect**—What key themes and recommendations were suggested by Jansen's research?

Sustainability vs. Self-Sufficiency

The term "sustainable" is used in many contexts, including health systems strengthening. Many projects are criticized as "unsustainable." The UN uses the word in its "Sustainable Development Goals, a blueprint for peace and prosperity for people and the planet, now and in the future." But what do we mean when discussing sustainable health services for the poor? Does that mean that the poor should pay for their healthcare? Does it mean that mission hospitals in low-income countries should not expect support from more prosperous nations to continue their work? Does it mean that healthcare programs should be "self-sufficient," somehow generating all the financial resources needed through fees that their services generate?

To be clear, healthcare for the poor can never be "self-sufficient" if it maintains even the most basic standard of quality. Quality care for the poor always requires resources that the poor simply do not have. While it is wise to build mechanisms for saving costs, improving efficiency, and generating income, "sustainable solutions" also include long-term partnerships for financial and other resources to initiate or maintain the work over a period of time.

Indeed, the Global church has a biblical responsibility to assure that the body of Christ looks after the needs of the whole body. Much as oxygenated blood moves from the lungs to the extremities, this should include the flow of resources from the enriched part of the body to where resources are needed the most. At the same time, the poor may have or develop non-tangible resources which contribute to sustainability, such as a knowledge of the local context, a love of neighbor flowing from a passion for Christ, and long-term endurance. The Word of God does not return void (Isa 55:11).

Minding the Gaps

As we examine health systems in developing countries (mainly Europe and the US), many of the most respected universities and hospitals were founded by local Christians responding to the greatest needs around them. Unfortunately, as these ministries became institutions, and as economic and social progress diminished, the greatest needs, some of them have lost the focus on serving the sick and the poor in the name of Christ. They were now too complex to be run by clergy and local believers and became professionalized. As professional organizations, rather than ministries, they became more focused on growing as influential and sustainable institutions rather than adhering to their original mission.

Who would Jesus seek to serve? Believers need to be aware of the vulnerable and the marginalized, providing equitable care for those who are part of the vision.

Some healthcare providers may have a particular passion for those on the streets, the drug addicted, the poor, and the refugees. Others work primarily in hospitals or institutions. Others work in community health and prevention. Strength comes from being motivated by Christ's heart, "filled with compassion for the lost sheep who were harassed and helpless and who did not know his name" (Matt 9:36).

Providing whole person care in a Christ-honoring way is a worthy goal for any faith-based hospital or health system. But the heart of Christ was not developing profitable health systems, nor was it simply to bring physical health and human flourishing. It was to bring freedom from the bondage of sin, to bring redemption to those made in God's image, to reconcile all of creation, and establish his kingdom on earth as in heaven. We have seen throughout the history of the church that mission is most transformational when it seeks to respond to gaps that the dominant society and systems inevitably leave. Globally, one of those gaps is intentional engagement with the unreached and unengaged people groups worldwide who have never heard the Name above All Names. Most of these groups also have a tremendous need for quality healthcare and prevention strategies.

Learning Activities

- **Read**—DeYoung and Gilbert, "What Is the Mission of the Church?: Making Sense of Social Justice, Shalom, and the Great Commission" (https://bit.ly/3SzD4ZS).

- **Reflect**—How can healthcare missions best navigate the balance between spiritual ministry and ministering to human needs? Is God calling you to fill this gap? What are some of the gaps you are aware of?

Part 5—Health Systems—Populations in Transition

Until the last century, global life expectancy was generally low by our standards (<40 years), and most people died from communicable diseases (or infections). Malaria, tuberculosis, and diarrheal illness were the leading causes of death. Therefore, healthcare missions are aimed first at treating infectious diseases and other prevalent conditions and eventually providing programs for preventing infections and transforming the health of the communities.

Improved health, and economic and social advancement, move together and impact each other. As countries become wealthier and more developed, health and life expectancy improve, especially where non-medical forces develop, such as general education, healthy family life, and character like Jesus outlined in the Sermon on the Mount. Countries trapped by conflict and corruption have been left behind and continue to suffer from poverty and disease.

Learning Activities

- **Watch**—Hans Rosling's "200 Countries, 200 Years, 4 Minutes— The Joy of Stats" (https://bit.ly/42f4dVg).

- **Reflect**—What are three ways you can use Dr. Rosling's information in your practice/ministry?

Some interesting patterns emerge as we examine changes in the cause and life expectancy over time and between countries. Social and economic advances lead to healthier environments, better healthcare services, and improved education, housing, water, and sanitation access. As a result, diseases like malaria, TB, and diarrhea dramatically decrease. Women are less likely to die in childbirth, and infants and children survive to adulthood.

In many of these societies, decreased premature death from preventable diseases is not the only thing that changes. People shift from rural to urban settings, from manual labor to desk jobs, and from growing their own food to eating cheap and highly processed foods. More stress, less exercise, and unhealthy living all contribute to increased risks for the "diseases of prosperity": hypertension, diabetes, heart disease, stroke, and many other "non-communicable" diseases (NCDs). This creates a "double burden" of disease in low- and middle-income countries.

The shift in disease and death from infectious diseases (usually at younger ages) to chronic, non-communicable diseases (usually at an older age) is referred to as the epidemiologic transition (NIH 2020). The epidemiological transition refers to changing population patterns related to data points such as morbidity, fertility, life expectancy, and mortality.

Learning Activities

- **Watch**—Martin, G. "Epidemiologic Transition" (https://bit.ly/47XFiqu).
- **Reflect**—What are the implications of these changes on the composition of populations in your context?

The epidemiologic transition and its contributing factors have a profound impact on the dynamics of the population. When early mortality is high, families tend to have many children to ensure that there will be an opportunity to have enough family to survive to carry on the family.

Historically, countries with high birth and death rates will have many young people, but the total *population can stay stable*. Countries with very low early death rates also tend to have low birth rates because aspirations for having children shifts from having "enough children to survive" to "wanting the best for each child" (education, vocational opportunities, etc.).

These countries can have flat or even negative population growth. **Population pyramids** are a valuable tool to visualize the proportion of the population at various ages. These dynamics also profoundly impact population growth. Early improvements in living conditions and interventions that address common communicable diseases will impact death rates. Still, it can take some time before the social norms shift to having fewer children. During this transition, these countries have rapid population growth.

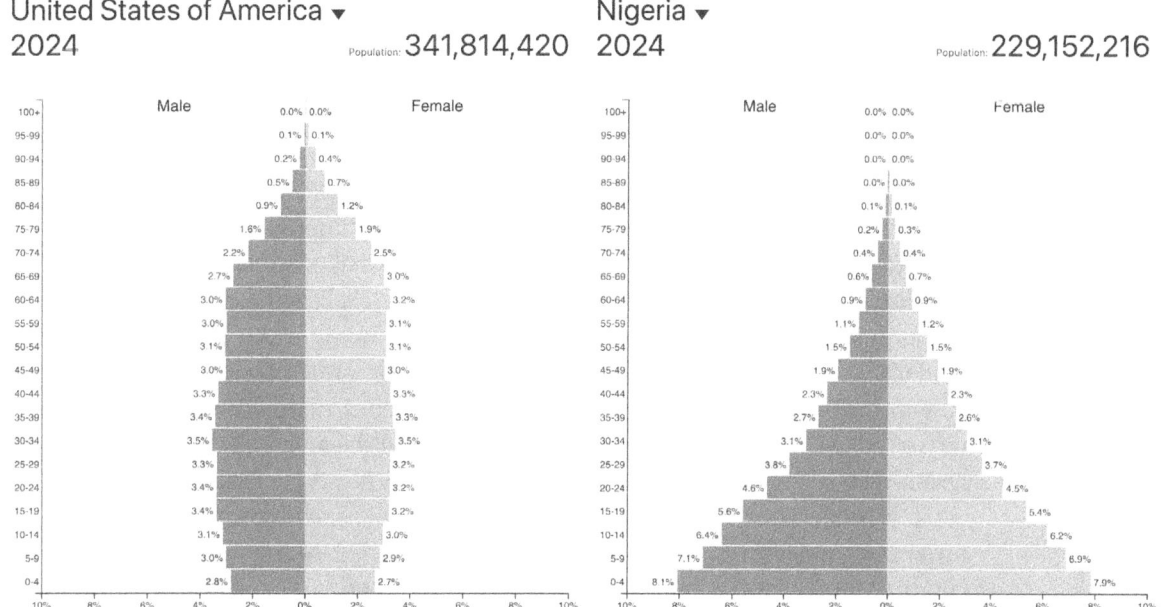

Figure 9: Population Pyramids of the World by Country from 1950 to 2100 (https://www.populationpyramid.net/world/2023/)

Learning Activities

- **Reflect**—How might these changes in demographics impact strategies for wholistic ministry in the future?
- **Reflect**—How might these changes in overall urbanization of the population impact wholistic ministry in the future?

Understanding Health Systems

The strategies discussed thus far exist within the larger context of healthcare systems. These healthcare systems exist within the larger context of historical, political, economic, social, and cultural factors contributing to health. In 2007, the World Health Organization (WHO) developed a framework for essential components of a health system that they call the Health System Building Blocks (see figure below). While it provides a helpful structure for understanding the multiple elements, it is an incomplete picture of the real-time functioning of complex health systems.

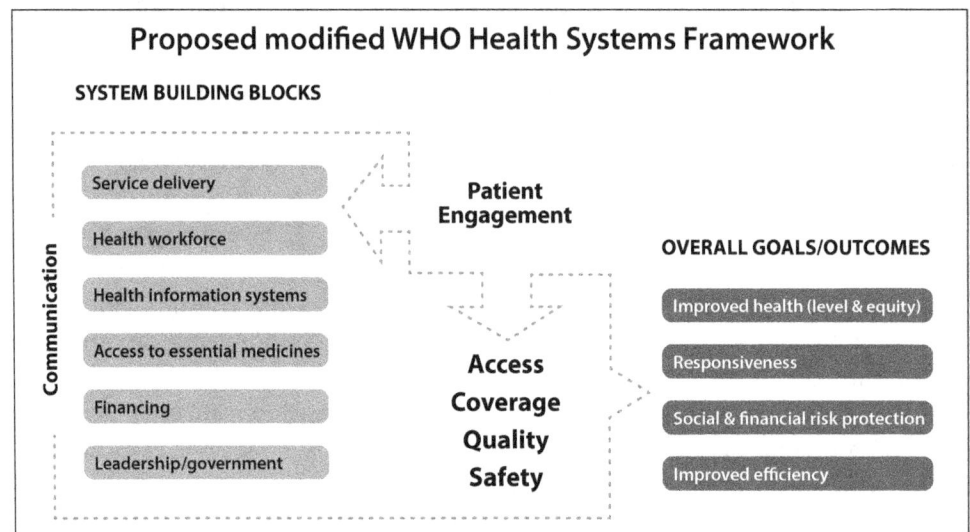

Figure 10: The WHO Health Systems Framework (https://healthsystemsglobal.org/news/a-new-era-for-the-who-health-system-building-blocks/)

This framework does not adequately include community and faith-based actor's critical role in healthcare systems. It also does not show complex interactions between these components and their relationship to the innumerable factors inside and outside the health system that impact health and healthcare service delivery.

Global Health Strategies and NGOs

Medical science, epidemiology and behavioral medicine, the spread of democracy, and improved living standards have all contributed to improved global health. Efforts are underway to create global health priorities, and goals have led to consolidated and coordinated efforts to impact some of history's most challenging diseases. Advances in vaccines, accompanied by strategies to distribute, and administer them, have saved countless millions of lives. In 2015, the UN identified a new set of development goals, called the Sustainable Development Goals (SDGs), that summarizes an agenda for the years leading up to 2030. SDG 3 is related to Good Health and Well-being for all and includes specific health-related targets, but each SDG impacts human health and well-being.

It is helpful for those involved in healthcare missions to be aware of and collaborate toward meeting shared goals for health. In general, the UN goals are not inherently in conflict with Christian values, but decisions around the implementation of programs addressing these goals need to include the voices of people of faith so that they protect religious freedom and honor the role of faith and faith institutions in healthcare.

The SDGs do not capture the larger context through which Christian's view health and well-being and its vital connection to the church as an integral part of the community.

Learning Activities

- **Watch**—United Nations. "Do You Know All 17 SDGs?" (https://bit.ly/47XFwOm).
- **Watch**—The Lancet's "Causes of Death: Global Burden of Disease Study 2015" (https://bit.ly/4bhwXB4).

These videos were created before the COVID pandemic, and since then, there has been a big shift in the secular world to deal with global health issues. In the past several decades, promoting human flourishing has shifted from being the work of the church and other faith-based institutions to an increasingly "professionalized" cadre of development organizations or non-governmental organizations (NGOs). These organizations often have full-time grants management staff and fundraisers; they have a definite advantage in competing for large grants in the development sector. This empowers them to document greater impact and return on investment from the donor's mindset. Because of changing policies in the US, faith-based organizations (FBOs) have been able to access resources previously dominated by NGOs. These FBOs have also demonstrated that they are not just a good return on investment but can also be critical to sustainable and locally relevant solutions.

Local vs. Autocratic Solutions

Increasing evidence demonstrates the importance of engaging local stakeholders in developing plans and priorities for development. Local stakeholders include the church when it exists. This requires recognizing that, while the donor has the money and the NGO/FBO has the tools, the community has the expertise to understand its needs and values. It also knows the history of what has and has not worked and who does and does not consider the benefit of the whole community.

Programs that tap into the creative power of local solutions and provide real-time feedback on the outcomes and impact of their work are more likely to be both contextually appropriate and sustainable. Donors and "experts" have their role in facilitating this process, but more often than not, the system promotes precisely the opposite; top-down, autocratic programs usually focus on measurable short- and medium-term goals and not on actual development. That which is truly good and sustainable in a community often flows out of seemingly insignificant efforts born out of the kingdom of God and the good news of the gospel.

Several development programs in the secular and faith-based sectors are taking an "Asset-based" approach to community development. Rather than evaluating what the community is lacking or failing to provide (a needs-based approach), the teams research the community and map the assets (people, organizations, facilities, resources, and programs) and then build upon these strengths, engaging them in planning and implementing and expansion of what they are already doing. This use of what can be termed "positive deviants" seeks out what those thriving in the same context are doing and not only taps into local resources, but maintains relational dignity, creates a balance of the donor-recipient relationship, and represents a more accurate reflection of the Body of Christ and *shalom*.

Learning Activities

a. **Watch**—"When Helping Hurts" (https://bit.ly/4bbm2IX).
b. **Reflect**—What are some ways we try to help that may not be helpful?

Systems Thinking in Global Health Mission

> But in fact, God has placed the parts in the body, every one of them, just as he wanted them to be. If they were all one part, where would the body be?
> (1 Cor 12:18–19)

Western thinkers, especially those in science and medicine, often employ methods of understanding that break down complex systems into their component parts, seeking an in-depth understanding. With this "reductionist" mindset, the practitioner aims to have a greater understanding of the "whole" by studying the component "parts." They seek to understand causality from a linear, cause-and-effect perspective. The reality is, however, that health problems and their root causes are far too complex to understand or intervene using such linear and reductionist thinking.

These settings represent a complex interplay of history, culture, values, and resources in a highly interconnected and interdependent network of individuals, communities, and institutions. These elements and interconnections are often invisible to the communities themselves, much less to outside visitors and missionaries. Understanding how these complex systems operate takes some deliberate study, reflection, and measured response.

Complexity vs Established Science

Complexity Science	Established Science
Wholism	Reductionism
Relationships among entities	Discrete entities
Non-linear relationships	Linear relationships
Quantum physics	Newtonian physics
Understanding, sensitivity	Prediction
Focus on variation	Focus on averages

Adapted from https://www.ncbi.nlm.nih.gov/pmc/articles/PMC2464825/.

New and growing disciplines of complexity science, network theory, and others have fostered an appreciation for such complex systems. They are beginning to help us understand how complex systems work and how they can be shaped. Often termed Systems Thinking, it describes "complex adaptive systems" and provides a new framework for viewing the "real-world systems" within which health-promoting Christ-followers exist, as well as insights into how to promote locally adapted innovations that apply the truths of Scripture, the work of the Spirit, and the expanding collective knowledge base.

Learning Activities

- **Watch**—"Simple Rules of Systems Thinking" (https://bit.ly/3HVjDF3). Note that there are some shorter versions you may choose to watch instead on YouTube.

- **Reflect**—Consider a current issue you are dealing with at work or in your personal life. Map out the Distinctions (people or principles), their Relationships, and how those form a System. Now reflect on the differing Perspectives that each brings to this issue. Does this provide additional insight on finding a "high leverage" solution?

- **Imagine**—Imaging how this map might be complete and more valuable if you had a diverse team thinking through these distinctions, relationships, and perspectives. If you can, try this with your team.

- **For Supplemental Reading**—Swanson and Thacker, "Systems Thinking in Short-Term Health Missions" (https://bit.ly/47QESlS).

Systems thinking clarifies that no one solution will work in every context, but rather that the best solutions arise from the "emergence" of local opportunities that work within the context of each unique system. Examining successful health programs with a "systems lens" has shed light on some principles of how these solutions arise. Watch the following video where Dr. Braithwaite outlines the lessons learned from a study in 60 countries.

Learning Activities

- **Watch**—Jeffrey Braithwaite's "Successful International Healthcare Reform" (https://bit.ly/3Sy6yrg).
- **Reflect**—Can you identify ways to apply these principles to your current work?

Bringing It All Together

There are many times in the Scriptures when the people of Israel faced new, seemingly insurmountable challenges. Leaders (Moses, Miriam, Aaron, Joshua, Deborah, Nehemiah, and others) retold the familiar story of God's miraculous interventions in the past to remind them of God's faithfulness and his ability to lead them through whatever was ahead. So far in this course, we have had a glimpse of how God has used healthcare missions in the past to build his church and bless his people, all to his glory. We have learned lessons about what works and what does not work through experience, research, and experimentation. Let us build upon this foundation as we seek to follow his lead for the future of global health mission.

References

Best Practices in Global Health Missions. (2021). Health Systems Strengthening and Health Topics. Project of Health for All Nations, https://bpghm.org/.

DeYoung, K., and Gilbert, G. (2011). *What Is the Mission of the Church? Making Sense of Social Justice, Shalom, and the Great Commission*. Crossway.

Gunderson, G. R., and Cochrane, J. R. (2012). *People Who Congregate: Building on Strengths.* In: *Religion and the Health of the Public*. Palgrave Macmillan, New York. 99–118 https://doi.org/10.1057/9781137015259_6.

Jansen, P. (2020). "Health Systems Strengthening Through Faith-based Sector: Critical Analysis of Facilitators and Inhibitors of Nationalization of Mission Hospitals in India." *Christian Journal for Global Health* 7(2): 104–19. https://journal.cjgh.org/index.php/cjgh/article/view/319.

Levin, J. (2014). "Faith-based Partnerships for Population Health: Challenges, Initiatives, and Prospects." *Public health reports* (Washington, D.C.: 1974), 129(2): 127–31.

McKeown, R. E. (2009). "The Epidemiologic Transition: Changing Patterns of Mortality and Population Dynamics." *American Journal of Lifestyle Medicine* 3(1): 19S–26S. https://doi.org/10.1177/1559827609335350.

Swanson, R. C., and Thacker, B. J. (2015). "Systems Thinking in Short-term Health Missions: A Conceptual Introduction and Consideration of Implications for Practice." *Christian Journal for Global Health* 2(1). https://doi.org/10.15566/cjgh.v2i1.50.

WHO. (2021). *Interventions on Diet and Physical Activity. What Works.* https://www.who.int/dietphysicalactivity/summary-report-09.pdf.

Reflection Questions for Group Discussion

DRSP Framework Review

- **Watch**—"Systems-Thinking: A Little Film about a Big Idea" (https://bit.ly/3vOGUFH).

- What are the four rules and their accompanying elements outlined in the DRSP framework for systems thinking?

_____(D)	_____(i)	_____(o)
_____(S)	_____(p)	_____(w)
_____(R)	_____(a)	_____(r)
_____(P)	_____(p)	_____(v)

Systems thinking clarifies that no one solution will work in every context, but rather that the best solutions arise from the "emergence" of local opportunities that work within the context of each unique system. Examining successful health programs with a "systems lens" has shed light on some principles of how these solutions arise.

Based on Dr. Braithwaite's lessons learned from a study in 60 countries (viewed above):

- **The Acorn to Oak Tree Principle**—Most projects start small and spread.
- **Data to Intelligent Principle**—Successful programs were able to translate mere data into intelligent information for decision making.
- **Starting with the Patient in Mind**—Successful programs begin with the patient at the center of the solution.

   a. What are three ways to apply these principles in your current practice and sphere of influence?

   b. Is there one principle that resonates more than another? Which one and why?

   c. Is there another method you use instead?

Be prepared to share your thoughts during facilitated group discussion.

Lesson 12
Leadership, Innovation, and Emerging Practices

Summary	Knowledge and Understanding Objectives
This lesson focuses on the way healthcare workers can model Christ-like leadership qualities which contribute to the church being ever more effective in reaching individuals, families, communities, and entire ethne with the gospel of Jesus the Messiah. This unique leadership style will also facilitate innovations at the frontier of missions so that more and more people groups know and follow Jesus.	1. Define and discuss what leadership has looked like in your own context. 2. Identify the leadership style modeled by Jesus and delineate why it is a better model. 3. Define and discuss your understanding of innovation. 4. Describe where you have seen innovation happen effectively in healthcare and the church.
Thematic Content	**Affective Objectives**
• The dominant leadership style in the world is typically a highly authoritarian model where non-leaders simply do as they are told. It is often based on fear of failure. • Christ-like leadership is counter-cultural. His was a leadership model based on humility and servanthood. • Adaptive leadership adjusts to the environment and its challenges, is culturally sensitive, and meets the needs expressed by those served. • Innovation is often misunderstood as being a new invention (the internet, smart phones, the personal computer, etc.). This is only partially the case. • Innovation to meet the overwhelming health/care needs of today will require a greater shift to servant leadership which is informed by the adaptive leadership model. • Best and emerging strategies are needed to implement the *Missio Dei*. • *Shalom* for all the families of the earth is the driving call.	1. Recognize and address your own leadership style that conflicts with a Christ-like leadership style. 2. Make the connection between humble, wholistic, Christ-like care of the individual, the family, and the community and *shalom*. 3. Demonstrate in your own calling to healthcare ministry, a Christ-like leadership commitment. 4. Acknowledge that innovations and strategies to address the complex global health challenges of our day will not occur because of individual effort but by involving key stakeholders, especially the communities for which you are serving. 5. Understand how sustainable community health is developed.
Conceptual Thread—Christ-like Leader	**Practice (Skills) Objectives**
The main goal of the leader is to serve and influence, as Jesus modeled for his followers. "Whoever wants to become great among you must be your servant, and whoever wants to be first must be your slave—just as the Son of Man did not come to be served, but to serve, and to give his life as a ransom for many" (Matt 20:26–28). "A Christ-like leader is … a person with God-given capacity and God-given responsibility who influences a group of followers toward God's purposes for the group" (Clinton 2012, 127)	1. Demonstrate Christ-like care and leadership in your own calling. 2. Serve toward a whole-person model of care for individuals and an integrated approach to community health, especially in populations where the gospel isn't known and/or health care is more limited. 3. Apply the concepts of Christ-like leadership and adaptive leadership in situations and challenges that are complex, and which require innovation.

Part 1—Leadership: Being a Person and a People of Influence

Christ-like Leadership

> You know that those who are regarded as rulers of the Gentiles lord it over them, and their high officials exercise authority over them. Not so among you. Instead, whoever wants to be first must be your servant, and whoever wants to be first must be slave of all. For even the Son of Man did not come to be served, but to serve and to give his life as a ransom for many. (Mark 10:42–45)

> Have this in mind among yourselves, which is yours in Christ Jesus, who, though he was in the form of God, did not count equality with God a thing to be grasped, but emptied himself, by taking the form of a servant, being born in the likeness of men. And being found in human form, he humbled himself by becoming obedient to the point of death, even death on a cross. (Phil 2:5–8)

It is within this biblical picture of servant leadership that Christ-centered healthcare takes its directives. The healing ministry of Jesus was clearly a servant-like and other-centered ministry. "And large crowds came to him, bringing with them those who were lame, crippled, blind, mute, and many others, and they laid them down at his feet; and he healed them" (Matt 15:30). The servant healing ministry of Jesus started with his Incarnation, was manifest in his life, death, and resurrection—setting a supreme example and ongoing presence in the church now and until his return. It is this Incarnational servant spiritual and healing ministry, which is key to whole-person health care and community-based ministry as we see from the life of Jesus. Further it is key to transformative multiplication of people, churches, and ministry.

Learning Activities

- **Read**—"What Is a Christ-Like Leader?" Lausanne Occasional Paper Section 5 (https://bit.ly/3u1kK2B).
- **Reflect**—What are the characteristics of Christ-like leaders you can implement?
- **Reflect**—How does your own culture or worldview see "servant leadership"? Is it seen as a negative attribute, a giving up of power or influence? How accurately does this reflect Christ's model of leadership?

Preparing the Heart to Serve

The Christ-like or servant-leader is a servant first. It begins with the Spirit-prompted willingness to serve followed by a conscious choice to lead. The best indication of success is that those served and led grow as persons. They become healthier, wiser, freer, more autonomous, more just, showing signs that they themselves are becoming servant-leaders. They show a particular concern for the least privileged or most vulnerable in society.

Christ-like character is the product of a life that is genuinely submitted to Jesus Christ and his word, just as Jesus the Son of God submitted to the Father. Leadership begins with *follower-ship*. The first step in the leadership development process for Jesus's disciples was to obey his call to "follow me." Only the one who has learned to follow is qualified to lead. Only the one who has learned to listen to God through meditation on the word of God and learning to recognize the promptings of the Spirit of God is prepared to speak for God. Submission requires humility and obedience.

The most important biblical principle for a Christ-like or servant-leader is love. This is not a love as the world knows it, but a love that puts God and neighbor first. It is a love that knows no limit to its endurance, no end to its trust, no fading of its hope; it can outlast anything. It is, in fact, the one thing that still stands when all else has fallen (1 Cor 13:7–8). This agape-like love shows itself in compassionate care for the whole person, especially those who are marginalized and/or suffering. "And when the Lord saw her, he had compassion on her and said to her, 'Do not weep'" (Luke 7:13). This was Jesus's response to a widow who had lost her only son.

Empathy is also important to develop in healthcare and global health ministry so that believers do not become mechanical or calloused to those they are called to serve. And this can only be a reality when those in ministry are skilled listeners.

According to Greenleaf (1977/2002 27), who is an expert in this area, the Christ-like or servant-leader includes at least these 10 characteristics which are derived from the example of Jesus's ministry:

- **Listening**—"Be quick to hear, slow to speak and slow to anger" (James 1:19). Listening is easy to talk about but hard to do but this is an indispensable character quality for leaders.

- **Compassion**—"And when the Lord saw her, he had compassion on her and said to her, 'Do not weep'" (Luke 7:13). This was Jesus's response to a widow who had lost her only son. Empathy is important to develop in the healing arts and not grow mechanical or calloused to those we are called to serve.

- **Healing (and Restoration)**—Though we cannot completely replicate the ministry model of Jesus we can show the healing and compassion of the Good Samaritan (Luke 10:25–37). Note Jesus's response to this story as to how to "Love our neighbors," was to, "go and do likewise" (Luke 10:37). We must work to continually develop wholistic healing and the skill of loving our neighbor sacrificially like Jesus. In like manner the fullness of Jesus's ministry focus is illustrated in the story of the woman with 12 years of bleeding in Luke 8:43–48 (paralleled in Mark 5:25–34). Not only did the woman receive physical healing but also healing of her mind, and spirit and was restored to her relationships with family and her community (*shalom*).

- **Awareness**—Jesus was at times crushed by crowds wanting to see and/or be healed by him. Jesus said when a woman with long term bleeding problems touched him, "Someone has touched me" (Luke 8:46). Though we may not know that power has gone from us like Jesus, we can feel depleted at times. We can learn to be aware of our surroundings and the prompting and power of the Holy Spirit to respond to people's needs. But we also must be aware of the need to take care of ourselves and renew our strength. Jesus demonstrated this from the outset of his ministry by getting away, alone with his Father at all hours of the night (Mark 1:35). Honoring the Sabbath is not a recommendation but a commandment!

- **Persuasion**—As leaders we will have to bring people together and empower them. "Jesus called his disciples together and gave them authority to drive out demons and to cure diseases and he sent them out to preach the kingdom of God and to heal the sick" (Luke 9:1–2). The ability to persuade came as he developed strong, non-coercive relationships with his disciples and then gave them specific requirements for going out to preach and heal (Luke 9:3–5). This should be the same for servant-leaders.

- **Conceptualization**—To conceptualize is really to see that which is not yet there but what can be in the future. Jesus was going through towns and was preaching and healing and had compassion on the people and said, "The harvest is plentiful, but the workers are few. Ask the Lord of the harvest to send out workers into his harvest" (Matt 9:35–38). Though Jesus as the Son of God had access to knowledge about the future, he was also the Son of Man and at times did not know all information. We can learn from Jesus how to conceptualize for a preferable future.

- **Foresight**—Foresight is having some insight into what might certainly happen. Jesus knew his message would bring opposition and he said so. "Be on your guard; you will be handed over to the local councils and be flogged in the synagogues" (Matt 10:17 NIV; but the whole passage of 10:5–42 addresses this issue in more detail). Jesus not only knew this through providential insight but given the normal response to the gospel and the news he was bringing. Leaders need this same type of foresight to give to their followers.

- **Stewardship**—This is not just ownership of resources but how they are managed. This is clearly addressed by Jesus in several parables (Luke 16:1–13) but Jesus's summary point was, "Whoever can be trusted with very little can also be trusted with much and whoever is dishonest with very little will also be dishonest with much." Stewardship is not just about money or buildings but also about the management of people.

- **Commitment to Growth of People**—The Apostle Peter finished out the second of his letters to a persecuted church by saying, "grow in the grace and knowledge of our Lord Jesus Christ" (2 Pet 3:18). The summary statement of these two letters is this: keep growing. It is leaders who keep this growth moving forward and multiplying.

- **Building Community**—All of the Epistles of the New Testament address this challenge of building community. The Apostle Paul addresses this clearly in his first book to the church in Thessalonica where he writes, "We always thank God for all the mentioning of you in our prayers" (1 Thess 1:2). Then later he states, "we loved you so much that we were delighted to share with you not only the gospel of God but our lives as well because you had become so dear to us" (1 Thess 2:8). Praying for those we are in community with and showing our love builds and is part of leading a community of grace.

When leaders are genuinely listening to God, and keeping in step with the Spirit of God, they will naturally find themselves in tune with one another as well. Jesus prayed that his followers would be one as the Father and Son were one, and that their complete unity would show the world that God loved them and had sent Christ (John 17:20–23). The proof to the world that the disciples were genuinely followers of Jesus would be their love for one another, the same love that Jesus had showed to them (John 13:34–35). The primary mark of the Christ-like leader, then, will be his/her love for other disciples of Jesus, including other Christian leaders.

The Christ-like leader doesn't settle for simple knowledge (Greek; *gnosis*) such as the fact that there are too few surgeons serving in Africa but seeks deeper knowledge (*epignosis*) which is also informed by greater understanding (*sunesis*) of the reasons behind the complex challenge being considered. This leads to wisdom (*sophia*) in how to act to overcome the challenge (Col 1:9 plus most all of Proverbs 1, which goes even deeper into these concepts). This will also equip the leader to better understand the times and cultures within which they are living and serving, fulfilling the role once practiced by the Sons of Issachar (1 Chr 12:32) who understood the times to know the best course for Israel to take.

In Hebrews 10:25, the author states:

> And let us not neglect our meeting together, as some people do, but encourage one another, especially now that the day of his return is drawing near.

But we are also living and participating in the larger system of our cultural context where we are called to be the salt and light that the world needs.

Adaptive Leadership

The world is a dynamic place and things are always changing. This means that believers must be aware of ways to navigate the changes as they lead others to the Lord and function within specific ministries. There are several models for leadership described by numerous authors, and they include authoritarian leadership, participative leadership, delegative leadership, transactional leadership, and transformational leadership. Adaptive leadership is a newer term, and it is an important idea to understand since cultures, languages, governments, and organizations differ in how they approach and communicate issues, challenges, problems and changes in their communities, villages, cities, and countries. It is important to develop knowledge, skills, the right heart, and even wisdom through adaptive leadership.

Adaptive Leadership and has been developed primarily through the research of Marty Linsky and Ronald Heifetz and is described in their book *The Practice of Adaptive Leadership*. One can become equipped in this model of leadership at the Kansas Leadership Center, which partnered with Marty Linsky to develop their programming. At the center of this leadership model is understanding the distinction between technical and complex/adaptive challenges. Also, you can understand these distinctions at a slightly deeper level by watching this brief video about the Cynefin Framework, (https://bit.ly/3OnxEPf).

Learning Activities

- **Read**—pages 4-9 in the Kansas Leadership Framework (dig deeper in the remaining pages if you choose) (https://bit.ly/3OkCSva).

- **Reflect**—what challenges are you called to confront most often?
  Are these mostly technical (simple/complicated) or adaptive/complex problems?
  The vast majority of the problems faced by healthcare workers in the context of the healthcare industry in the West are either simple or perhaps complicated (as per the Cynefin Framework).

- **Write**—Based on the diagram on page 6 of the KLC book, list 5 of the most common problems you are tasked with dealing with and list them as either technical or complex/adaptive. List at least 3 complex/adaptive challenges you can think of that the global church is facing with regards to seeing people amongst all nations experiencing fullness of life and good health.

- **Read**—Acts 1:3-8. Reflect on how the disciples had to demonstrate adaptive leadership.

Jesus was a master at adapting to rapid changes and challenges to his work and ministry, although being fully human, and fully divine, he already knew when the need to adapt would occur. His followers can look at the ways he adapted and navigated change. He knew when to stay and when to leave. He knew how to ask key questions to those opposing him and challenged those he worked with daily to improve their leadership skills, so that when he was gone, they were able to carry on his work and ministry. Jesus was constantly challenged and even attacked by people, but he avoided being trapped in order to accomplish the Father's plan.

One example of this was when Jesus was asked about paying taxes to Caesar (Luke 20:20–26) and the resurrection and marriage (Luke 20:27–40). When asked, "who is my neighbor?" Jesus responded with the story of the Good Samaritan (Luke 10:25–37). The disciples, however, had to learn how to adapt and be flexible with changes. In the following passage (Acts 1:3–8) how did the disciples have to demonstrate adaptive leadership?

> After his suffering, he presented himself to them and gave many convincing proofs that he was alive. He appeared to them over a period of forty days and spoke about the kingdom of God. On one occasion, while he was eating with them, he gave them this command: "Do not leave Jerusalem, but wait for the gift my Father promised, which you have heard me speak about. For John baptized with water, but in a few days, you will be baptized with the Holy Spirit." Then they gathered around him and asked him, "Lord, are you at this time going to restore the kingdom to Israel?" He said to them: "It is not for you to know the times or dates the Father has set by his own authority. But you will receive power when the Holy Spirit comes on you; and you will be my witnesses in Jerusalem, and in all Judea and Samaria, and to the ends of the earth."

Part 2—Innovation

If there is one word that most people have a foggy understanding of it would be innovation. There may be as many definitions of the word innovation as there are for leadership. It is likely that most would function from a mental model that understands innovation to mean things like the personal computer, the light bulb, and the internet as great innovations. Were those innovations? Yes. But those would better be classified as inventions rather than innovations. But is this the only viable understanding of innovation? No, it is not. Cormode (2020) explains in his book about innovation that Christian innovation occurs when believers make spiritual sense of the situations in their lives. He focuses on three things:

1. Mental models come to believers as stories, and they dictate behavior.
2. Christian tradition comes as a series of beliefs which need to be recalibrated around contemporary expressions.
3. Christian innovation is the innovation of meaning—and how that allows believers to reinterpret ancient practices (often by changing mental models).

Let's focus on the last one of the elements, innovation of meaning, while keeping in mind all three. Cormode identifies at least five types of innovation:

1. Product innovation—Adapting therapies, tools, and interventions for better efficacy.
2. Process innovation—Creating new ways to deliver services or reach preferred outcomes.
3. Internet innovation—Facilitating communication via new apps and websites.
4. Social innovation—Pursuing change in the name of a social value by "social entrepreneurs" who take direct action to transform the existing system.
5. Innovation of meaning—Worldview perspectives renewed and reformed based on "cultural entrepreneurship."

The first four types of innovation noted above depend largely on the concept of creative destruction which means it is also disruptive and discontinuous. This would imply innovation that involves replacing one thing with another (better) thing, be it a device, a process, or a social system. This tends to establish a belief that the past must be abandoned to make progress a reality. Not all processes and practices are bad or need to change, and some may just need to be improved to meet current needs. A thorough assessment will ensure that if completely new ways to deliver services, for example, are needed, they are done from a biblical perspective.

Cormode (2012) goes on to discuss the fact that innovation is not a new thing, but rather a new way of seeing things, and perhaps a way to use the good practices of the past in a new way. He gives two examples of this type of innovation that occurred in the church: one being the example of Martin Luther and the Reformation and the second being Ralph Winter's insight as to the meaning and understanding of the word "nations" (*ethne*) in Scripture.

Learning Activities

- **Reflect**—on your own calling to health-related ministry work (this includes pastors caring for their people) and
- **Identify and list**—at least three places where you can see "systems" (including the church) that are clinging to old mindsets that might be inhibiting innovations in health-related ministry from happening. With the Adaptive Leadership model in mind, list 3 ways you might become involved in influencing at least one of these systems toward innovation that doesn't seek to break away from the past but instead harnesses the past in powerful ways.
- **Watch**—"Innovation Is about Connection" by Andrew Hargadon (https://bit.ly/47UAbaG). What does he identify as a key component of innovation?

Part 3—Effective Strategies and Emerging Practices

This lesson has presented some new ideas about leadership and innovation. But these will not lead to transformation if they do not honor God and do not contribute to human health and flourishing (*shalom*), and unless there is action taken by God's people to address the root cause of human disease and suffering. If believers have identified a complex challenge, believe they are being called to overcome, and if they have utilized the adaptive leadership principles then they will end up with potential solutions which could become innovations.

Doing this requires that all those involved understand that failure may be a frequent companion and that it is acceptable. Entrepreneurship and innovation require taking risks. For example, if a person comes up with ten experiments to try and nine fail but one succeeds, then that is called success. But taking risks and accepting some failures is not a common element of most cultures. It will be a huge but important calling to work in this sphere of ministry.

There is not space in this lesson nor in this course to delve into moving from idea to actual implementation. However, we recommend exploring the website of the D School at Stanford, https://dschool.stanford.edu/, or the company website for IDEO https://www.ideo.com/, both of which use the concepts of design thinking to create innovations in diverse fields. Briefly, design thinking is an approach to generate creative solutions and can include a) empathizing with the end-users; b) defining the problem from their point of view (vulnerability); c) ideating solutions (imagining); d) creating a prototype of those solutions; and e) testing the solutions with the people with the problem and in the context where the problem occurs.

What we will do here, at the end of this lesson, is look at some examples of effective strategies in the past and present to creatively lead others toward health, healing, and wholeness among the nations. We will return to Jesus, the author and perfector of our faith.

Learning Activities

Study Mark 1:16–39—Within a very short period of time (Mark uses "immediately" quite often) Jesus gave a very clear demonstration of the most important aspects of his earthly ministry. Dr Fountain used to describe this incident as the first recorded whole-person community health clinic open to all in the history of the world at the time.

- Preaching/proclamation (vv. 14, 15) Jesus **proclaims** in this passage, "The time is fulfilled, and the kingdom of God is at hand, repent and believe in the gospel."
- **Discipleship** (vv. 16–20)—having disciples/followers was common for rabbis at the time. But this was a unique kind of discipleship. They were to follow and fish for people!
- **Teaching** (vv. 21–22)—this was not unusual in the synagogue setting. It was where teaching was expected, but his was unique. **In what way?**
- **Deliverance** (vv. 23–27)—**what was innovative about this element of Jesus's ministry?**
- **Healing** (vv. 29–34)—physical healing. Was this unique at the time? The Greek word used in verse 34 is *etherapeusen*, which means "healed, reversing a physical condition to restore a person having an illness (disease, infirmity)" (Strongs). Many of the afflicted were drawn toward the disciples (v. 33), and multiplied service and mission were outcomes of healing (v. 31).
- Going to the people (vv. 35–39)—**what were Jesus's priorities at this point?** Jesus could have simply set up shop in Capernaum and let the world come to him to address their felt need for healing.
- But he chose to go to the people to preach—where they lived and worked and suffered. In like manner we can set up clinics and hospitals as places for the suffering masses to come to be healed, but we must also go where they are and enter their context with a message of deliverance and fullness of life and health.

There are many different strategies to address health care issues either in more developed or less developed countries or regions. It is important to keep in mind the goal of *shalom*, which has already been presented. It is also important to keep a kingdom of God mindset as his reign is applied to every aspect of embodied life in community. This is key in being able to implement a gospel ministry, which develops the best health outcomes in the short and long term throughout the world.

Accessible and quality health care is not the ultimate end of what we do as believers in Christ, though an important part of witness to the Divine Healer. What is important is that those we serve find reconciliation with God, grow as obedient disciples into a mature faith in Christ, hold out hope for abundant and eternal life in Jesus to others, and engage the world with acts of loving service, as healing agents in the context of the church.

Leadership, Innovation, and Emerging Practices

Learning Activities

- **Read**—Fountain, "Effective Strategies for Health" in *Health the Bible and the Church*, Ch. 15, 197–216 (https://bit.ly/3PvzApp).
- **Reflect**—Write your thoughts about unique ways to use each of these strategic approaches:
    1. Wholeness
    2. Integration
    3. A Team Approach
    4. A Community Approach
    5. Multiplication
    6. Education for Health and Wholeness
- **Watch**—"The Mayoko Story" (https://vimeo.com/125726852).
- **Explain**—the mindset shift Dr Fountain made after the little boy was brought back to the hospital by his mother a second time.

Part 4—Complex/Adaptive Challenges and Priorities

There is a myriad of health-affecting etiologies in both the material world and the spiritual realms which often overlap as covered in Lesson 2. Tracing these helps identify priority issues for Christian (transformational) health development and relief services. Approaching global health challenges with biblically informed solutions is an exercise of discernment and stewardship.

Vulnerable Populations

What is a vulnerable population? A vulnerable population or individual may have less perceived power, resources, and access, due to environmental, psychosocial, or physiological factors. This may result in being at greater than average risk of developing health problems. Examples are war and drought which cause vulnerability among populations and result in different issues to address. Families without fathers, people with mental illness, disenfranchised ethnic minorities, the poor, the displaced, the elderly, women, children (especially during gestation and early childhood), and the disabled may be the most vulnerable. Malnutrition can contribute to vulnerability and be chronic in some societies, directly affecting the health and well-being of whole nations.

As Christians the Scriptures are clear about our responsibility to care for those who are oppressed, poor or marginalized. For example, Isaiah 61:1–2 begins to outline the mission of Jesus as Messiah, which started to be fulfilled in his hometown in Nazareth (Luke 4:14–21).

> The Spirit of the Lord God is upon me,
> Because the Lord has anointed me to bring good news to the afflicted;
> He has sent me to bind up the brokenhearted,
> To proclaim liberty to the captives and freedom to prisoners,
> to proclaim the year of the Lord's favor.

Health Disparities

Health disparity refers to a higher burden of illness, injury, disability, or mortality experienced by one group relative to another. Healthcare disparity typically refers to differences between groups in health insurance coverage, access to and use of care, and quality of care.

Identifying the health disparities between wealthy (high-socio-demographic index, SDI) countries and poor (low-SDI) countries does not tell the whole story. Disparities in health are also quite evident between the rich and the poor within most countries. India has become a destination for what is called "medical tourism" because it can offer first-world care at a fraction of the cost in the US or other western countries. Yet, throughout India, the poor are still not able to access even basic primary healthcare services. Health outcomes in the US vary depending upon ethnicity, socio-economic class, level of education, language, ability or disability, age, family context, and other factors. In every country, there is a dramatic disparity in access to healthcare services between urban and rural communities. These healthcare disparities represent gaps that the church should be aware of and respond to.

Environmental and Planetary Health

This content could be a whole lesson in itself, and it does tie back to the first few lessons on the biblical basis for mission. It is important to consider environmental health because it impacts human health in so many ways. According to the WHO (2016), all the physical, chemical, and biological factors around us need to be examined so balance and optimal health can occur. Environmental concerns such as air pollution, carbon emissions, climate change, ozone depletion, water pollution, deforestation, energy depletion, unhealthy foods, and waste disposal cause significant effects to health and well-being.

When the Alma Ata Declaration was written, global health leaders recognized there were healthcare disparities and global trends that needed to be changed. This eventually led to other global health initiatives across the world. The Sustainable Development Goals emphasized the interdependence of human well-being with planetary flourishing. With the increasing interconnectedness across the globe, health issues today are more universal, and ever-changing. We saw this connectedness play out with the COVID epidemic that turned into a pandemic and is now endemic.

Health Promotion and Disease Prevention

Health promotion and disease prevention (HPandP), presented in Lesson 10, include innovative actions that are designed to foster a healthy lifestyle and a safe environment. There are three categories of disease prevention from a public and community health perspective. Primary prevention includes interventions that occur before health effects occur and diseases develop. Secondary prevention includes screening measures used to detect and treat disease at its earliest stages before the onset of signs and symptoms.

Tertiary prevention focuses on managing disease after diagnosis, by trying to limit disability for those with incurable disease and includes rehabilitation to prevent further deterioration and enhance functionality. Disease prevention and health promotion are important aspects of Primary Health Care, and the most cost-effective measure to promote health in communities. Healthcare workers who focus on disease management and rehabilitation are an important part of this continuum of prevention; they add value through compassionate care, which builds trust and gains entrance for healing conversation and dialogue.

Public Sphere and Advocacy for Justice

> On my account you will be brought before governors and kings as witnesses to them and to the Gentiles. (Matt 10:18)

All Christ-followers have a responsibility to "... *act justly and to love mercy and to walk humbly with your God*" (Micah 6:8). Health workers have a unique platform of influence, not just by compassionate care to individuals, influence life-promoting behavior, and interact with those in power. A Christian health worker's role is not only treating illness and sharing the gospel, but also using their influence to advocate for policies that protect the vulnerable and promote community health and well-being.

Speaking truth to power, strengthening health systems, and advocating for those who are subject to injustice is participating in the work of Jesus as servants in his kingdom. Pastors and other church leaders can also be advocates for those who are subject to injustice, and if both the medical side and the spiritual side of wholistic care occurs, restoration to *shalom* will be the result.

Multiplication

Multiplication in the pure sense means more rapid increase than simple addition. For example, if we were to build a house a month that would be twelve in a year. But if we build one a month, and each new homeowner builds one each month, and so on, there would be 2,048 houses at the end of that year. That is multiplication.

What does this mean in the context of Christian health-related ministries? It is very clear that Jesus healed hundreds if not thousands by simply touching them as a sign of the coming kingdom. He commissioned first his 12 apostles, then the 72 disciples to preach and heal (Luke 9:1–6; 10:1–9). Then toward the end of his earthly ministry, he said, "whoever believes in me will do the works I have been doing, and they will do even greater things than these, because I am going to the Father" (John 14:12). He believed in training, empowerment, and multiplication. Jesus's extensive investment in his disciples allowed for the church's rapid multiplication of not just new disciples but churches. Though marred by sin and subject to death, human beings (body and soul) who "live and believe" in every nation are given a sure hope of a resurrected body at Jesus's return (1 Cor 15). Thus, the healing ministry of Jesus was expected to extend beyond his time on the earth and be magnified throughout all the earth, and into eternity.

Priority in the Least Reached Places

Jesus commissioned his disciples to make disciples among all ethno-linguistic people groups on earth (Greek *ethne*. Matt 28:18–20). Yet today, there remain 7,400 (depending on how it's measured) people groups who have little access to meeting Christ-followers or hearing the gospel (<2% evangelical, <5% Christian adherent). Moreover, 1.94 billion people, or 1 in 4 on the planet, live in frontier people groups (<0.1% Christian) and have no access to the gospel message. Most of these live in what is known as the "10/40 Window." Many of these disproportionately suffer significant health challenges. "Least reached" could mean most deprived of resources, health services, and/or the presence of a thriving church.

Outreach efforts in these high priority areas of the world must mold their efforts into the form of ministry Jesus demonstrated to the world. It was a whole person ministry that served the mind, body and spirit of the person in the context of their family and community. Examples exist in the present day of healing work done in this mold that have contributed to the planting of God's kingdom within previously unreached and unengaged (frontier) people groups.

The Great Divide

One of the most interesting problems that has puzzled many in the mission community is the ongoing gap that exists between those desiring to plant churches in unreached people groups and those doing wholistic care outreach. The two groups seem to speak different languages and circulate in different worlds. They rarely understand how essential they are to each other. There seems to be a chasm between healthcare ministries, church planting movements (CPM), and disciple making movements

(DMM), as all these ministries attempt to reach the unreached peoples of the world. There needs to be more of an emphasis on ways to bridge the divide for a collaborative, unified movement.

Part of this divide occurs because many do not have a full understanding of the kingdom of God. They function from the kingdom of Salvation paradigm (or mindset). The latter tends to think all the church needs to do is get people saved from their sins. While this is surely a major reason for the incarnation, life, death, and resurrection of Jesus, it is not all there is to it. People become part of the kingdom of God to engage in the battle against the works of Satan. This spiritual battle was discussed in Lesson 9 and includes things such as witnessing to the powers and principalities, as well as fighting disease, disasters, suffering, and death.

A close connection exists between the Word of God going forth, healing of the nations, and restoration of *shalom*. Healing was the context which preceded the Sermon on the Mount (see Matthew 5). The advance of that kingdom is visible when the church, the body of Christ, serves to restore and comfort those with physical, spiritual, and mental concerns in the context of living in a broken world. The long view of the kingdom continues with every "*tribe, language, people and nation*" before the Lamb (Rev 7:9), having access to the leaves of the Tree of Life for healing of the nations (Rev 22:1–3).

To the Ends of the Earth

Throughout the previous lessons, the idea that God has called his people to join him on mission, the *Missio Dei*, and all that he is doing in the world has been emphasized. The task is not just to heal, to make disciples, and plant churches in all the geopolitical places of the world, but rather to reach, make disciples, baptize, and teach *panta ta ethne* (all the nations)—all the ethnolinguistic people groups of the world with his word. Christ-followers receive power from the Holy Spirit, and there is no limit to sharing his word for the health, wholeness, and healing of all peoples—restoring *shalom*.

Believers are to be his witnesses, wherever the Lord has them serving, and no matter what their profession may be. In the book *Preach and Heal*, Chuck Fielding clarifies a significant point on this subject that the healing and preaching ministry of the church go hand-in-hand like two handles of a plow (2006). Believers have this example in Luke to proclaim his kingdom and to heal:

> He called the twelve together and gave them power and authority over all demons and to cure diseases, and he sent them out to proclaim the kingdom of God and to heal. And he said to them, "Take nothing for your journey, no staff, nor bag, nor bread, nor money; and do not have two tunics. And whatever house you enter, stay there, and from there depart. And wherever they do not receive you, when you leave that town shake off the dust from your feet as a testimony against them." And they departed and went through the villages, preaching the gospel and healing everywhere. (Luke 9:1–6)

Therefore, in the ministry of the gospel, preaching and wholistic health and healing go hand-in-hand. Proclamation of the gospel is tied closely with demonstration by word and deed, with each member of the church exercising their respective gifts and talents.

> "But you will receive power when the Holy Spirit has come upon you, and you will be my witnesses in Jerusalem and in all Judea and Samaria, and to the ends of the earth" (Acts 1:8).

References

Clinton, R. (2012). *The Making of a Leader: Recognizing the Lessons and Stages of Leadership Development.* NavPress.

Cormode, S. (2020). *The Innovative Church: How Leaders and Their Congregations Can Adapt in an Ever-Changing World.* Grand Rapids, MI: Baker Academic.

Fielding, C. (2006). *Preach and Heal: A Biblical Model for Missions.* Richmond, VA: International Mission Board.

Fountain, D. (1989). *Health, the Bible, and the Church.* Billy Graham Center.

Healthy People 2000. Modified for 2010, 2020, and Now 2030. https://health.gov/healthypeople.

Levin, J. (2014). "Faith-based Partnerships for Population Health: Challenges, Initiatives, and Prospects." *Public Health Rep.* 129(2): 127–31.

WCC (1964. 1965). *World Council of Churches: The Healing Church. The Tübingen Consultation* Geneva (World Council Studies 3).

World Health Organization—WHO (1978). *Health for All by the Year 2000.* Alma Ata Declaration. https://www.who.int/.

World Health Organization—WHO (2016). Environmental and Planetary Health. https://www.who.int/.

Reflection Questions for Group Discussion

Read Psalm 67 and reflect on the meaning

1. How does Psalm 67 relate to the biblical foundation for mission?

2. What will cause the nations to rejoice according to the verses?

3. How does one build and multiply the kingdom, bringing the nations to an understanding of the one true God?

4. How is our common understanding of "nations" different than a biblical understanding of ethne or every tribe, language, people, and nation (Rev 7:9)?

5. Describe 3 ways you can advocate for the poor and marginalized and pursue justice (Micah 6:8).

Contributors

Arnold Gorske (MD, FAAP) is the CEO of Standards of Excellence in Healthcare Missions and the editor for Health Education Program for Developing Communities. He is a member of the CHIM governance team, Best Practices in Global Health Missions Working Group, and various Christian health mission boards. He is part of the HFAN leadership team and served as medical team leader for the International Red Cross in Iraq, followed by over fifty short-term missions to numerous countries worldwide.

Christoffer H. Grundmann (ThD, Dr. Theol. habil) is the John R. Eckrich University Professor in Religion and the Healing Arts at Valparaiso University, Valparaiso, Indiana, USA. He teaches courses on missiology and comparative religions, and his research includes topics related to medical missions, healing, medicine of the person, and corporeality. He has authored numerous publications, including the book *Sent to Heal! The Emergence and Development of Medical Missions*.

Paul Hudson (MD) is a missionary physician and epidemiologist who served with SIM in Ethiopia, Nepal, and Thailand for over thirty years. Service areas include clinical medicine, community health, discipleship, and the intersection of faith and practice. Paul spent about half his medical missionary career with SIM globally, developing gospel-based approaches to HIV and AIDS and coaching medical missionaries on three continents. He has written about connections between healthcare and the gospel in *Healthcare and the Mission of God*.

Perry Jansen (MD, MPH, DTMH) has twenty years of experience as a clinician, manager, and strategist in sub-Saharan Africa. He is the Vice President of Strategic Health Partnerships with African Mission Healthcare and has also worked with other sending agencies. He considers himself a systems thinker and appreciates the complex adaptive systems people work in. He is an encourager and catalyzer for local solutions for the next generation of healthcare leaders.

Rebecca Meyer (PhD, MSNed, BSN, RN) has been a nurse for over thirty-five years, working in the PICU/CVICU as part of the ECMO Team and Transport Team and as an Educator, Charge Nurse, and Manager. A full-time professor since 2010, she served as the curriculum coordinator and co-author of Christian Global Health in Perspective, part of Health for All Nations. She trains and leads students to serve cross-culturally and integrate their faith with their discipline.

Daniel O'Neill (MD, MTh) is a physician-theologian and managing editor of the *Christian Journal for Global Health (cjgh.org)*. He is the author and co-editor of the book *All Creation Groans: Toward a Theology of Disease and Global Health* (Pickwick, 2021). He has served on multiple health and development projects in Latin America, India, Burkina Faso, and the Middle East. He is an Assistant Clinical Professor of Family Medicine at the University of Connecticut School of Medicine.

Mike Soderling (MD, MBA) served as an OB/GYN physician in a multi-specialty group in the US for ten years before following a call to Central America, where he served for eleven years. He is the Director of Health for All Nations, seeking to see people from every tribe, tongue, and nation experience the health/shalom of Jesus.

Grace Tazelaar started out teaching nursing education at a diploma school and was involved in its transition to a baccalaureate program. She left nursing education to do community health development in Uganda from 1985 to 1991. It was at the end of the civil war and the beginning of the HIV/AIDS pandemic. Her career focus changed from women's health to public health during that time. After the war, she worked with the Ministry of Health and the Ministry of Education as they developed the first baccalaureate nursing program in the area. Grace now serves as the NCF Missions Director in a volunteer role.

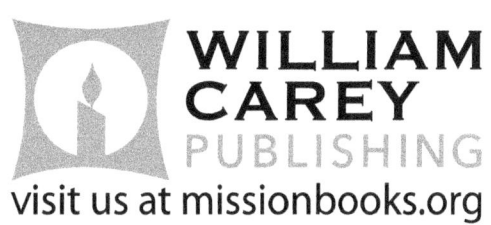

visit us at missionbooks.org

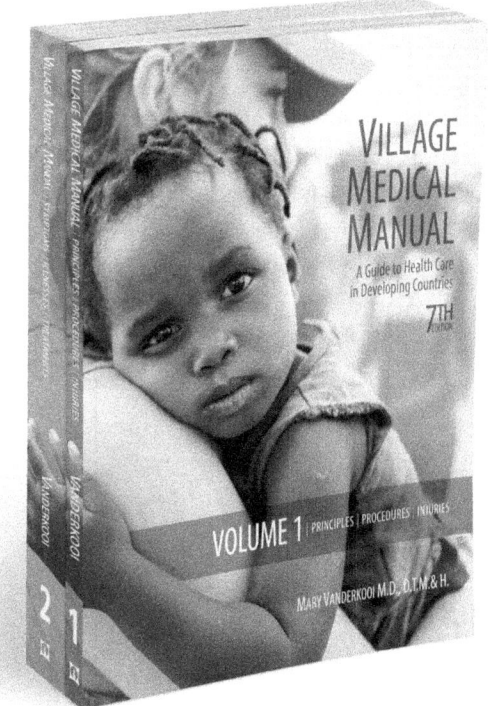

Village Medical Manual: A Guide to Health Care in Developing Countries (7th ed.)

Mary Vanderkooi, M.D., D.T.M.& H.

Village Medical Manual is a user-friendly, two-volume healthcare guide for lay workers in developing countries with special features that trained medical professionals would also find useful. Its intended use is for those who are required, by location and circumstances, to render medical care.

The clear vocabulary, along with over a thousand illustrations and diagrams, help Western-educated expatriates living in isolated locations to medically treat people and intelligently refer those that can be referred accordingly. It contains clearly defined procedural techniques and diagnostic protocols for when sophisticated instrumentation and lab tests are not available. It also offers solutions and advice for overcoming barriers to best practices in global health.

Volume 1: Principles, Procedures, and Injuries elucidates medical principles, symptoms, and procedures for routine medical care, as well as emergency situations.

Volume 2: Symptoms, Diagnosis, and Treatment includes vast symptom, disease (common and tropical), drug, and regionally-relevant indices to assist the reader in step-by-step diagnoses and treatment.

This is a crucial reference for all who lack formal global health training but must know how to meet health care challenges in developing areas lacking medical infrastructure.

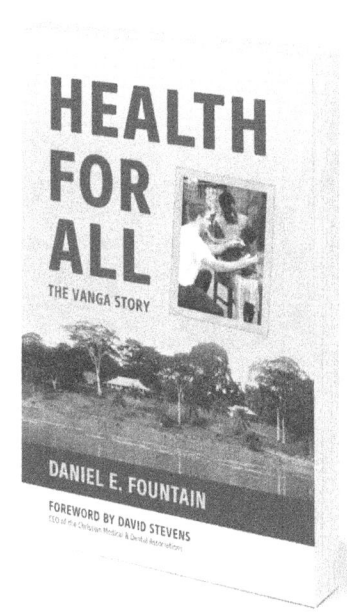

Health for All: The Vanga Story

Daniel Fountain

When Dan Fountain and his wife arrived in the Congo in 1961, the challenges to effective medical missions seemed overwhelming. As the only doctor for a quarter of a million residents of the Vanga Health Zone, and with nothing but a dilapidated mission hospital and an undertrained staff to run it, Dr. Fountain turned to prayer, innovation, and local partnerships to meet the vast needs of his area.

Health for All tells the story of an ever-increasing vision—from curative care to community health, from a barely functioning hospital to a network of successful health services, from a lack of qualified workers to a local residency training program, from biomedical reductionism to whole person care, from cultural stalemate to worldview transformation. Part memoir, part history, part textbook, *Health for All* is the legacy of a man who patterned his life and labor after that of the Great Physician.

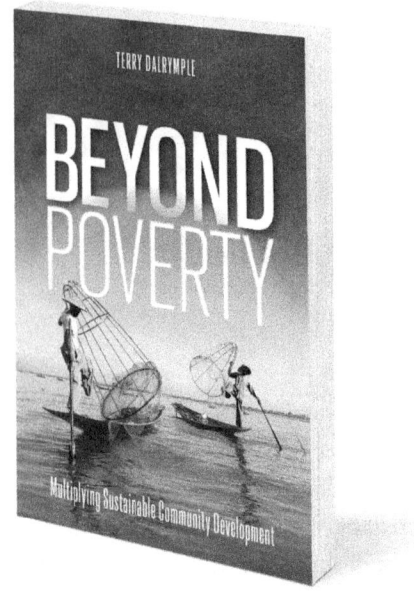

Beyond Poverty: Multiplying Sustainable Community Development

Terry Dalrymple

The church is facing a strategic opportunity—85 percent of people living in extreme poverty around the world reside in villages. In *Beyond Poverty*, Terry Dalrymple calls us to move beyond sustainable projects in a single village to transformational movements that multiply change from village to village and sweep the countryside.

Through multiple case studies based on the actual experiences of more than 900 organizations in 135 different countries, this book tells the story of a large and growing network of ministries around the world using the strategy of Community Health Evangelism to change the life of the poor forever. The principles in this book are not just a theory, but proven strategy. This book will help you understand the fundamentals of catalyzing transformational movements that make disciples among the poor while lifting whole communities out of cycles of poverty and disease.

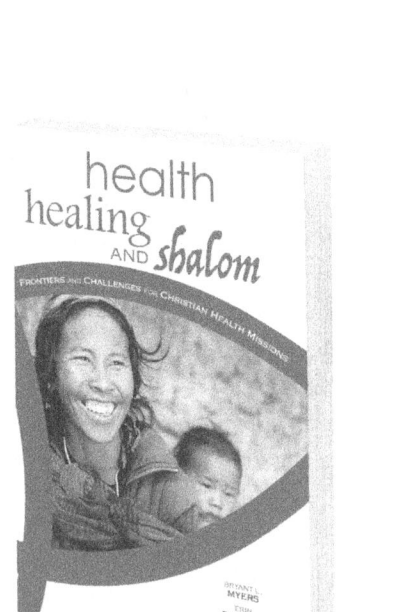

Health, Healing, and Shalom: Frontiers and Challenges for Christian Healthcare Missions

Bryant L. Myers, Erin Dufault-Hunter, Isaac B. Voss, editors

In this edited volume, authors with an interest in health missions from a wide variety of experiences and disciplines examine health and healing through the theological lens of shalom. This word, often translated "peace," names a much more complex understanding of human well-being as right relationships with one another, with God, and with creation. Reading various aspects of healthcare missions through these glasses not only yields much-needed correctives to current practice but also exposes the Spirit's invitation to participate in God's ongoing work of tending, caring, and healing our broken world.